Socio-Affective Computing

Volume 7

Series Editor
Amir Hussain, University of Stirling, Stirling, UK

Co-Editor
Erik Cambria, Nanyang Technological University, Singapore

This exciting Book Series aims to publish state-of-the-art research on socially intelligent, affective and multimodal human-machine interaction and systems. It will emphasize the role of affect in social interactions and the humanistic side of affective computing by promoting publications at the cross-roads between engineering and human sciences (including biological, social and cultural aspects of human life). Three broad domains of social and affective computing will be covered by the book series: (1) social computing, (2) affective computing, and (3) interplay of the first two domains (for example, augmenting social interaction through affective computing). Examples of the first domain will include but not limited to: all types of social interactions that contribute to the meaning, interest and richness of our daily life, for example, information produced by a group of people used to provide or enhance the functioning of a system. Examples of the second domain will include, but not limited to: computational and psychological models of emotions, bodily manifestations of affect (facial expressions, posture, behavior, physiology), and affective interfaces and applications (dialogue systems, games, learning etc.). This series will publish works of the highest quality that advance the understanding and practical application of social and affective computing techniques. Research monographs, introductory and advanced level textbooks, volume editions and proceedings will be considered.

More information about this series at http://www.springer.com/series/13199

Ranjan Satapathy • Erik Cambria • Amir Hussain

Sentiment Analysis in the Bio-Medical Domain

Techniques, Tools, and Applications

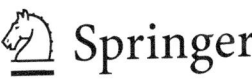 Springer

Ranjan Satapathy
School of Computer Science & Engineering
Nanyang Technological University
Singapore, Singapore

Erik Cambria
School of Computer Science & Engineering
Nanyang Technological University
Singapore, Singapore

Amir Hussain
Division of Computing Science
University of Stirling
Stirling, UK

ISSN 2509-5706   ISSN 2509-5714 (electronic)
Socio-Affective Computing
ISBN 978-3-319-88609-1   ISBN 978-3-319-68468-0 (eBook)
https://doi.org/10.1007/978-3-319-68468-0

Printed on acid-free paper

This Springer imprint is published by Springer Nature
The registered company is Springer International Publishing AG
The registered company address is: Gewerbestrasse 11, 6330 Cham, Switzerland

This book is dedicated to my father Mr. Prabhakara Satapathy whose hard work, sacrifices and motivational speeches have led me to where I am and my mother Mrs. Anima Satapathy who has been keeping things sorted in my life.

Preface

The opportunity to capture the opinions of the general public has raised growing interest both within the scientific community, leading to many exciting open challenges, and in the business world due to the remarkable range of benefits envisaged, including from marketing, business intelligence and financial prediction. Mining opinions and sentiments from natural language, however, is an extremely difficult task as it involves a deep understanding of most of the explicit and implicit, regular and irregular and syntactical and semantic rules appropriate of a language. Existing approaches to sentiment analysis mainly rely on parts of text in which opinions are explicitly expressed such as polarity terms, affect words and their co-occurrence frequencies. However, opinions and sentiments are often conveyed implicitly through latent semantics, which make purely syntactical approaches ineffective.

Natural language processing (NLP) has been used to address a wide range of problems including support for search engines, summarizing and classifying text for web pages and incorporating machine learning technologies to solve problems such as speech recognition and query analysis. NLP is used to enhance the utility and power of applications. It does so by making user input easier and converting text to more usable forms. The usable forms include lexicons like WordNet, WordNet for Medical Events (WME), Medical FactNet (MFN), Medical BeliefNet (MBN) and Medical WordNet (MWN).

This book focuses on the applications of sentiment analysis in the biomedical domain and combining computational creativity and machine learning. The applications include building a medical lexicon with the aim of supporting experts and non-experts in the medical field. The main aim of this book is to bridge the gap between the industrialists and the academicians working in the field of biomedical text mining. It is the need of the hour for both worlds to work together towards achieving their common goal. This book will bring both the experts' interest into a common platform. This book focuses on explaining the research gaps, in biomedical domain, namely:

1. Bridging the gap between the patients' and experts' multidimensional way of expressing their symptoms and diseases. The book introduces different scenarios where the problem lies and tries to solve the gaps by introducing a lexicon for biomedical domain.
2. Introducing a novel approach to combine computation creativity and machine learning to find the best 'K' for K-means clustering on WME dataset.

Singapore, Singapore   Ranjan Satapathy
Singapore, Singapore   Erik Cambria
Stirling, UK   Amir Hussain
June 2017

Acknowledgements

I would like to express my gratitude to Dr. Vineet C.P. Nair, Professor, University of Hyderabad. Your precious scoldings will always keep me pushing to work hard and make you proud!

I would also like to express my special appreciation to Dr. Amir Hussain and Dr. Erik Cambria for motivating me to write this book and supporting me through their valuable comments during the proofreading of this book. Last but not the least, I extend my thanks to the faculty members, my classmates and juniors of the University of Hyderabad.

Contents

List of Contributors

Ranjan Satapathy School of Computer Science and Engineering, Nanyang Technological University, Singapore, Singapore

Erik Cambria, PhD, Assistant Professor School of Computer Science and Engineering, Nanyang Technological University, Singapore, Singapore

Amir Hussain, PhD, Professor Division of Computing Science, University of Stirling, Stirling, UK

Acronyms

AI	Artificial intelligence
ANN	Artificial neural network
ANEW	Affective Norms for English Words
BACK	Benchmark for affective commonsense knowledge
CF-IOF	Concept frequency–inverse opinion frequency
CLSA	Concept-level sentiment analysis
DAUs	Daily active users
ELM	Extreme learning machine
FMRI	Functional magnetic resonance imaging
GWAPs	Games with a purpose
GECKA	Game engine for commonsense knowledge acquisition
HCI	Human-computer interaction
IV	In vocabulary
JL	Johnson-Lindenstrauss
KB	Knowledge base
MAUs	Monthly active users
MFN	Medical FactNet
MBN	Medical BeliefNet
MWN	Medical WordNet
MediConceptNet	Medical concept network
MDS	Multidimensional scaling
NLP	Natural language processing
OOV	Out of vocabulary
OMCS	Open Mind Common Sense
PAM	Partitioning Around Medoids
PCA	Principal component analysis
POS	Part of speech
POG	Prerequisite-outcome-goal
RP	Random projection
RPGs	Role play games
SMS	Short message streams

SRHT	Subsampled randomized Hadamard transform
TM	Text mining
TMN	Text message normalization
TSVD	Truncated singular value decomposition
VZIG	Varicella zoster immune globulin
WME	WordNet for Medical Events
WNA	WordNet-Affect

List of Figures

List of Tables

Chapter 1
Introduction

Abstract This introductory chapter reviews the general area of sentiment analysis research and posits a case for incorporating commonsense knowledge in machines, as a means to better understand natural language. In particular, the chapter introduces converging paradigms of sentiment analysis and biomedical text mining. Subsequently, a comprehensive literature review of commonsense knowledge representation is presented, together with a discussion on why commonsense is required for sentiment analysis and natural language understanding. Next, the chapter introduces computational creativity and concepts of computation and medical lexicons. Finally, the chapter concludes with a brief discussion of key challenges involved in sentiment analysis.

Keywords Opinion mining • Sentiment analysis • Biomedical text mining • Natural language processing • Deep learning • Computational creativity

As humans have developed language(s) to communicate with one another, so we need to make machines understand human language so as to communicate with them. In order to do that, machines need to interact with humans in their daily life and learn, how they talk and respond to situations. For that, we need data points, so as to make machines learn how to respond to different situations. Situations are represented as data points. Humans make use of past data by adapting themselves to different scenarios from the experiences of the past. Fortunately, for researchers data is abundantly available over the internet. Since 2003, there has been a huge increase in the unstructured data due to the increasing use of the internet. As this data is unstructured so direct machine translation is not possible. The unstructured data need to be converted into structured one so that it is understood by humans and machines. Until now, online information retrieval, aggregation, and processing have mainly been based on algorithms which rely on the textual representation of web pages. These algorithms' capabilities are limited when it comes to interpreting the input sentences and extracting meaningful sentences out of it. Today, most

© Springer International Publishing AG 2017   1
R. Satapathy et al., *Sentiment Analysis in the Bio-Medical Domain*,
Socio-Affective Computing 7, https://doi.org/10.1007/978-3-319-68468-0_1

of the algorithmic approaches still rely hugely on co-occurrence of words. *These algorithms can only process that information that they can see.* When it comes to humans, every word in a text activates a network of semantically related concepts, relevant episodes, and sensory experiences: which helps in completion of complex NLP tasks. To make machines more intelligent we need to make them work and think like humans which need to be trained on the huge amount of data.

The opportunity to capture the opinions of the general public has raised growing interest both within the scientific community and in the business world (data analytics field). However, mining sentiments and opinions from natural language (text or speech), is an extremely difficult task as it involves the deep understanding of the syntactic and semantic of that particular language or form. Current approaches involve searching for *explicit polarity terms, affect words* and *their co-occurrence terms.* However, in most of the cases, opinions and sentiments are often conveyed implicitly. Until now, online information retrieval, aggregation, and processing have mainly been based on algorithms relying on the textual representation of webpages. Such algorithms are very good at retrieving texts, splitting them into parts, checking the spelling, and counting the words. However, when it comes to interpreting sentences and extracting meaningful information, their capabilities are known to be very limited.

Early works aimed at classifying entire documents as containing overall positive or negative polarity, or rating scores of the reviews. Such systems were mainly based on supervised approaches relying on manually labeled samples, such as movie or product reviews where the opinionist's overall positive or negative attitude was explicitly indicated. However, opinions and sentiments do not occur only at document-level, nor they are limited to a single valence or aspect. Contrary attitudes towards the same topic or multiple topics can be present across the span of a document. Later works adopted a segment-level opinion analysis aiming to distinguish sentimental from non-sentimental sections, e.g., by using graph-based techniques for segmenting sections of a document on the basis of their subjectivity, or by performing a classification based on some fixed syntactic phrases that are likely to be used to express opinions. In more recent works, text analysis granularity has been taken down to sentence-level, e.g., by using the presence of opinion-bearing lexical items (single words or n-grams) to detect subjective sentences, or by exploiting association rule mining for a feature-based analysis of product reviews. These approaches, however, are still far from being able to infer the cognitive and affective information associated with natural language as they mainly rely on knowledge bases that are still too limited to efficiently process text at sentence-level. Moreover, such text analysis granularity might still not be enough as a single sentence may contain different opinions about different facets (aspects) of the same product or service.

This chapter covers topics which include common tasks in web mining in Sect. 1.1, sentiment analysis in Sect. 1.2, computational creativity in Sect. 1.3, introduction to biomedical text mining in Sect. 1.4 and discusses the problems of sentiment analysis in Sect. 1.5 and concludes with the brief introduction to deep learning.

1.1 Common Tasks in Web Mining

The Web is evolving towards an era where communities will define future products and services [25]. In this context, public opinion is destined to gain increasing prominence, and so are affective computing and sentiment analysis (see Fig. 1.1). The basic tasks of affective computing and sentiment analysis [2] are emotion recognition and polarity detection. Although the former focuses on extracting a set of emotion labels, the latter is usually a binary classification task with outputs such as "positive" versus "negative", "thumbs up" versus "thumbs down", or "like"

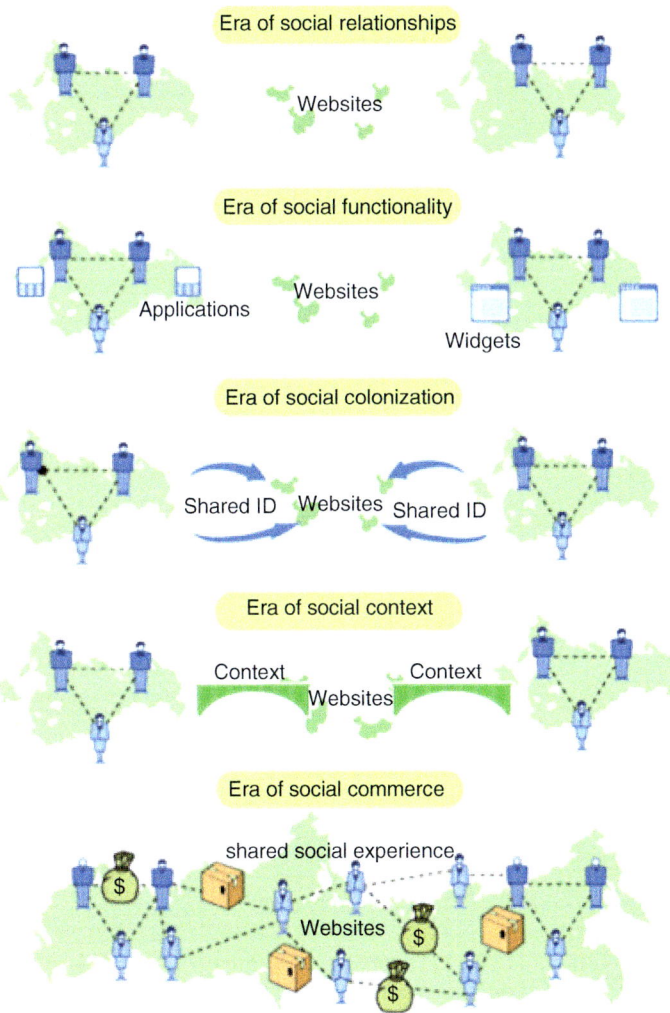

Fig. 1.1 The 5 eras of the Web vision (Source: [2])

versus "dislike". These two tasks are highly interrelated and interdependent to the extent that some sentiment categorization models, such as the Hourglass of Emotions [4], treat them as a unique task by inferring the polarity associated to a sentence directly from the emotions this conveys.

In many cases, in fact, emotion recognition is considered a subtask of polarity detection. Polarity classification itself can also be viewed as a subtask of more advanced analysis. For example, it can be applied to identify the pro and con expressions that can be used in individual reviews to evaluate the judgments on a product thereby making such judgments more trustworthy. Another instance of binary sentiment classification is agreement detection, that is, given a pair of affective inputs, deciding whether they should receive the same or differing sentiment-related labels. Complementing the binary sentiment classification is the assignment of degrees of positivity to the detected polarity or valence to the inferred emotions. If we waive the assumption that the input under examination is opinionated and is about a single issue or item, new challenging tasks arise, such as subjectivity detection and opinion target identification [6]. The capability of distinguishing whether an input is subjective or objective, in particular, can be highly beneficial for a more effective sentiment classification. Moreover, a record can have a polarity without necessarily containing an opinion – for example, a news article can be classified as *good* or *bad* news without being subjective. Typically, affective computing [29] and sentiment analysis are performed over on-topic documents (for example, on the result of a topic-based search engine). However, several studies suggested that managing these tasks jointly can be beneficial for overall performance. For example, off-topic passages of a document could contain irrelevant affective information and misleading results for the global sentiment polarity about the main topic. Also, a document can contain material on multiple topics that might interest the user. In this case, it is, therefore, necessary to identify the subject and isolate the opinions associated with each of them.

1.2 Sentiment Analysis

Sentiment Analysis [7] aims at determining the attitude of an author or a speaker with respect to some topic or the overall contextual polarity of a document. The attitude may be his or her judgment or evaluation, the emotional state of the author while writing (affective state), or the intended emotional communication (in other words, the emotional effect the author wishes to have on a particular reader or a group of reader intended). This section (Sect. 1.2) discusses the sentiment analysis in general and describes the different approaches to sentiment analysis in Sects. 1.2.1 and 1.2.2. A basic task in sentiment analysis is classifying the polarity of a given text at the document, sentence, or aspect-level – whether the expressed opinion in a document, a sentence or an aspect is positive, negative, or neutral. Advanced, "beyond polarity" sentiment classification looks, for instance, at emotional states such as "angry", "sad", and "happy". Early works in sentiment analysis area include

Turney [41] and Pang [28] who applied different methods for detecting the polarity of product reviews and movie reviews respectively. This work was focused on the document level. One can also classify a document's polarity on a multi-way scale, which was attempted by Pang [27] and Snyder [34] among others: Pang and Lee expanded the basic task of classifying a movie review as either positive or negative to predicting star ratings on either a 3 or a 4 star scale, while Snyder [34] performed an in-depth analysis of restaurant reviews, predicting ratings for various aspects of the given restaurant, such as the food and atmosphere on a 5-star scale. Even though in most statistical classification methods, the neutral class is ignored under the assumption that neutral texts lie near the boundary of the binary classifier, several researchers suggest that, as in every polarity problem, three categories must be identified. The importance of Neutral Class in Sentiment Analysis and the SVMs [15] can benefit from the introduction of a neutral class and improve the overall accuracy of the classification. There are in principle two ways for operating with a neutral class. Either, the algorithm proceeds by first identifying the neutral language, filtering it out and then assessing the rest in terms of positive and negative sentiments, or it builds a three-way classification in one step [32]. The second approach often involves estimating a probability distribution overall categories (e.g., Naïve Bayes classifiers as implemented by Python's NLTK[1] kit). Whether and how to use a neutral class depends on the nature of the data: if the data is clearly clustered into neutral, negative and positive language, it makes sense to filter the neutral language out and focus on the polarity between positive and negative sentiments. If in contrast, the data is mostly neutral with small deviations towards positive and negative affect, this strategy would make it harder to clearly distinguish between the two poles.

A different method for determining sentiment is the use of a scaling system whereby words commonly associated with having a negative, neutral or positive sentiment with them are given an associated number on a Likert scale [33] (most negative up to most positive). This makes it possible to adjust the sentiment of a given term relative to its environment (usually at sentence level). When a piece of unstructured text is analyzed using natural language processing tools, each concept in the specified environment is given a score based on the way sentiment words relate to the concept and its associated score [37]. This allows movement to a more sophisticated understanding of sentiment because it is now possible to adjust the sentiment value of a concept relative to modifications that may surround it. Words, for example, that intensify, relax or negate the sentiment expressed by the concept can affect its score. Alternatively, texts can be given a positive and negative sentiment strength score if the goal is to determine the sentiment in a text rather than the overall polarity and strength of the text [38]. There are many works [5] trying to address the problem of automatic sentiment analysis using machine learning. There are two major tasks in the sentiment analysis. The first one being *sentiment detection*, which classifies the text into subjective or objective sentences [26]. The

---

[1]http://www.nltk.org/

second task is *polarity classification*: given a piece of text with an opinion, the goal is to classify the sentiment to one of two polarities, i.e., positive or negative. These two tasks can be done on different levels, and there are different techniques for different level as well: n-gram and lexicon are usually used on term level while Part-of-Speech works for sentence and phrase analysis. Fundamentally, sentiment classification starts with identifying the semantic orientation of words, then goes to higher level text structure like the semantic orientation of sentences and documents. Several techniques are used to achieve this task: words were directly weighted by lexicons of semantic words which were manually or automatically constructed.

The performance of polarity classification could decrease if the model considers traditional bag-of-words features which may include some misleading texts. Most of the manually constructed lexicons are extensions of the general-purpose ones. In addition, a variety of training data labeled manually could help to perform supervised sentiment classification. Manual labeling is a tedious job and getting domain experts to get the job done is even more difficult. Utilizing contextual information could help depending less on human experts and makes our model automated. It also helps to increase the accuracy of sentiment analysis significantly. Therefore, the popular algorithms in machine learning, such as support vector machines and Naïve Bayes, are used to train the sentiment classifier. Meanwhile, by simply combining the polarities (summing it together) of all words, a document can only have two possible polarities, and no extreme opinion exists. Besides the two extreme polarities i.e., positive and negative category, mixed opinions are classified by introducing threshold values in identification. The main motive of sentiment analysis task is to make machines think more like humans. What if computers would be able to do what humans are capable of; feel what humans need; think human-like? The most important difference between traditional Artificial Intelligence (AI) systems and human intelligence is human's ability to harness commonsense knowledge gleaned from a lifetime of learning and experiences to enrich our decision-making and behavior. This allows humans to adapt easily to novel situations where AI fails catastrophically for lack of situation-specific rules and generalization capabilities. Humans are able to process unstructured data to structured data because of the ability to connect the words at the semantic level. The years of experience comes into account for these scenarios.

While to the average person the term commonsense is regarded as synonymous with good judgment whereas to the AI community, it is used in a technical sense to refer to the thousands of basic facts and understandings possessed by most human being, e.g., *"Sugar is sweet"*, *"To write a code, you must switch on your PC first"*, *"if you forget to wish your mother on mother's day, she may be unhappy with you"*. In order to better understand and interact with the people around us, we need to incorporate all the facts about them which we term as commonsense. Commonsense knowledge is what we learn throughout our lives and what we are taught about the world we live in during our initial years. Commonsense has no universal definition, rather it is more cultural and context dependent. Despite the language barrier, however, moving to a new place involves facing habits and situations that might go against what we consider basic rules of social interaction (commonsense) or things we were taught by our parents, such as "eating with chopsticks", "eating from someone else's plate", "handshaking when you meet a person", "slurping on noodle-like food or while drinking tea", "eating on the street", "crossing the road despite the heavy traffic", "squatting when tired", "removing shoes before entering home", "talking loudly with your friends on the streets" "growing long nails in the baby fingers", or "bargaining before you buy anything". This can happen also the other way round, that is when you do something perfectly in line with your commonsense that violates the social norms, e.g., "cheek kissing as a form of greeting" or "bowing down and saying namaste when you meet new people as a form of greeting" Machines, which never had the chance to live a 'human-like' life, have no commonsense at all and, hence, know nothing about us and our social norms. To help us work, computers must get to know what our jobs are and how we work. To entertain us, they need to know what we like and/or dislike. There has been significant evidence that rational learning in humans is emotional. To take care of us, machines need to know how we feel. To understand us, they must think as we think. However, today the actual scenario, in fact, is that computers do only what they are programmed to do. The very first person to think about the creation of a machine which could think was perhaps Alan Turing way back in 1950. He was the first to raise the question "Can machines really think? [40]". Whilst, he could never manage to answer that question, he provided the pioneering method to gauge AI, which we know it as *Turing test*. The notion of commonsense in AI actually dates back to 1958, when John McCarthy, in his seminal paper *"Programs with Commonsense"*, proposed a program, termed it as an "advice taker". It used to solve problems by shaping sentences in a formal language. The main aim of such a program was to try to automatically deduce for itself a sufficiently wide class of immediate consequences of anything it was asked from what it already knew. In his paper, McCarthy stressed the importance of finding a proper method of representing expressions in the field of computer science; since, according to him, in order for a program to be capable of learning something, it must first be capable of being told. He also developed the idea of creating a property list for each object, in which the specific things people usually know about that object are listed. It was the very first attempt to build a commonsense knowledge base but, more importantly, his work inspired the vision for a need of commonsense to move forward in the technological evolution.

The next Sect. 1.2.1 discusses the subjectivity and objectivity identification. As mentioned earlier, it is a method of detecting the neutral class at an earlier stage which makes polarity classification as a binary classification problem.

1.2.1 Subjectivity and Objectivity Identification

This task is defined as classifying a given text (sentence or tweet) into one of the two classes: objective or subjective. Objective sentences are the ones with neutral polarity including the factual information as well. Subjective sentences are the sentences which carry opinions i.e., either positive or negative. This problem is more difficult than polarity classification [23]. The subjectivity of words and phrases depends on their context and an objective document may contain subjective sentences (e.g., a news article quoting people's opinions). Moreover, as mentioned by Su [36] results are largely dependent on the definition of subjectivity used when annotating texts. However, Pang in [26] showed that removing objective sentences from a document before classifying its polarity helped improve performance. Authors in [8] proposed a Lyapunov deep neural network which outperforms baselines by over 10% and the features learned in the hidden layers improve our understanding subjective sentences in Spanish. In this paper, authors consider using a Lyapunov linear matrix inequality to classify Spanish text as subjective or objective by combining Spanish features and features obtained from the corresponding translated English text. Similarly, in [9], authors proposed a bayesian network based extreme learning machine model for subjectivity detection.

The next Sect. 1.2.2 discusses the Aspect identification. As mentioned earlier, it is a method of detecting the aspect a text is talking about.

1.2.2 Feature/Aspect Identification

Aspect identification [21, 31] refers to determining the opinions or sentiments expressed on different features or aspects of entities, e.g., of a cell phone, a digital camera, or a bank [11]. A feature or aspect is an attribute or component of an entity, e.g., battery of a mobile phone, the ambiance of a restaurant, or sound quality of an earphone. The advantage of feature-based sentiment analysis is the possibility to capture nuances about objects of interest. Different features can generate different sentiment responses, for example, a smartphone can have a great display, but lacks good battery backup. This problem involves several subproblems, e.g., identifying relevant entities, extracting their features/aspects, and determining whether an opinion expressed on each feature/aspect is positive, negative or neutral [20]. The automatic identification of features can be performed with syntactic methods or with topic modeling [39, 43]. Further detailed discussion can be found in Liu's work [17].

1.2.3 Different Resources for Sentiment Analysis

Sentiment vocabularies and annotated word lists:

1. Affective Norms for English Words (ANEW)
2. SenticNet [5]
3. SentiWordNet
4. WordNet-Affect
5. Emoji Sentiment Ranking

Online sentiment analyzers:

1. 30 dB[2] (free)
2. AlchemyAPI[3] (commercial)
3. Aylien[4] (free and commercial)
4. BitextAPI[5] (commercial)
5. Etuma Oy[6] (commercial)
6. HPE Haven OnDemand[7] (commercial, with freemium)
7. Semantria[8] (commercial)
8. Sentiment140[9] (commercial, for Twitter)
9. Stanford NLP [35] (academic)
10. Sentic API[10] (academic)
11. Twinword[11](commercial, free/unlimited)
12. Werfamous[12] (free)
13. WordStat[13] (commercial)

1.3 Computational Creativity

Section 1.3.1 gives an insight into creativity and concepts of computations Sect. 1.3.2 in AI. In this field, scientists probe whether machines can be made as creative as humans. And if yes, how to incorporate creativity and in what form.

1.3.1 What Is Creativity

According to [1];

Creativity is the ability to come up with ideas or artifacts that are new, surprising, and valuable.

---

[2]http://www.30db.com

[3]http://www.alchemyapi.com

[4]http://aylien.com/sentiment-analysis

[5]https://www.bitext.com

[6]http://www.etuma.com

[7]https://dev.havenondemand.com/apis/analyzesentiment#overview

[8]www.semantria.com

[9]www.sentiment140.com

[10]http://sentic.net/api

[11]www.twinword.com

[12]www.werfamous.com

[13]www.provalisresearch.com

Unfortunately, novelty, surprise, and value are not only difficult to define objectively as they also overlap. For instance, an idea rarely is surprising or valuable if it is not novel. Human creativity is something of a mystery, not to say a paradox. One new idea may be creative, while another is merely new. What's the difference? And how is creativity possible? Creative ideas are unpredictable. Sometimes they even seem to be impossible – and yet they happen. How can that be explained? Could a scientific psychology help us to understand how creativity is possible? Creativity is the ability to come up with ideas or artifacts that are new, surprising and valuable. 'Ideas' here include concepts, poems, musical compositions, scientific theories, cookery recipes, choreography, jokes – and so on. 'Artefacts' include paintings, sculptures, steam engines, vacuum cleaners, pottery, origami, penny whistles – and many other things you can name. As these very diverse examples suggest, creativity enters into virtually every aspect of life. It's not a special 'faculty' but an aspect of human intelligence in general: in other words, it's grounded in everyday abilities such as conceptual thinking, perception, memory, and reflective self-criticism. Hence, it isn't confined to a tiny elite: everyone of us is creative, to a degree.

1.3.2 Concepts of Computation

Our daily lives depend to a great extent on maps. There are maps, and there is map-making. A map can be incomplete in many different ways: a village omitted, a river misplaced, the contours too coarse-grained to help the wanderer. However, inadequate maps do not show map-making to be a waste of time, and clumsy contours do not prevent 'contours' from being a useful concept. Furthermore, map-making is an incremental process. They improve, as cartographers' geographical knowledge increases and think up new ways of charting it. However, a map is a map, even without Mercator's projection or lines of latitude. In short, if we want an efficient description of our landscape, map-making is a relevant activity.

Likewise, there are computer programs, and there are computational concepts. If current programs fail to match human thoughts, it does not follow that the theoretical concepts involved are psychologically irrelevant. Indeed, many of these concepts are more precisely-defined versions of psychological notions that existed years before AI came to the rescue. Moreover, AI researchers are as creative as anyone else. New computational concepts and new sorts of a program are continually being developed. Even while you are reading this book, there are researchers developing something new. For instance, neural network systems illuminate combinational creativity much better than early AI did. This is a new science, barely half-a-century old.

However, AI can provide dynamic processes as well as abstract descriptions. Consequently, it can help us to compare generative systems clearly and to test the computational power of individual heuristics in specific problem-solving contexts. The 'dynamic processes', of course, are functioning computer programs. A program together with an appropriate machine is what computer scientists call an effective procedure. An effective procedure need not be 'effective' in the sense of succeeding in the task for which it is used: doing addition, recognizing a harmony, writing a sonnet. All computer programs are effective procedures, whether they succeed in that (task) sense or not. An effective procedure is a series of information manipulating steps which, because each step is unambiguously defined, is guaranteed to produce a particular result. It can include a sum of integers if a particular step in the program instructs the machine to add the integers in the list; but the following step must specify what is to be done next, depending on which number happened to be picked. Given the appropriate hardware, the program tells the machine what to do and the machine can be relied upon to do it.

One example where computation creativity is constantly improving is 'music'. Western music springs from a search space defined by the rules of harmony and its melodies are pathways through a precisely mappable landscape of musical intervals. There are rules about musical tempo, too, which define a metrical search-space. An acceptable melody (a series of notes that is recognizable as a tune) must satisfy both rule-sets – perhaps with some tweaking at the margins. However, these rules, though intuitive, are not self- evident. Adding rules, in this case, is an incremental process. It requires the knowledge of music and programming both.

The next Sect. 1.4 introduces to the Biomedical text mining. Like Computational Creativity, Biomedical text mining also requires the knowledge of domain and programming. Domain knowledge helps to put down rules whereas programming helps to make it automated.

1.4   Biomedical Text Mining

Biomedical text mining also known as Bio-NLP refers to text mining applied to texts and literature of the biomedical and/or molecular biology domain. It is a research area at the edge of natural language processing, bioinformatics, medical informatics and computational linguistics. One common application of text mining is event extraction, which encompasses deducing specific knowledge concerning incidents referred to in texts. Event extraction can be applied to various types of written text, e.g., online news messages, blogs, and manuscripts. Text mining techniques are employed for various event extraction purposes [10]. It provides general guidelines on how to choose a particular event extraction technique depending on the user, the available content, and the scenario of use.

Text Mining (TM)[14] is concerned with information learning from preprocessed text (e.g., containing identified parts of speech or stemmed words). By means of text mining, often using Natural Language Processing (NLP) techniques [22], information is extracted from texts of various sources, such as news messages and blogs, and is represented and stored in a structured way, e.g., in databases. A specific type of knowledge that can be extracted from the text by means of TM is an event, which can be represented as a complex combination of relations linked to a set of empirical observations from texts (Fig. 1.2).

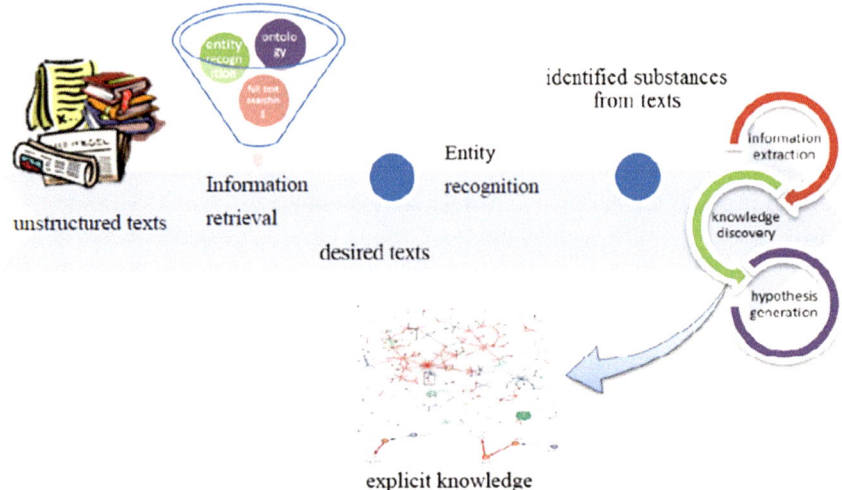

Fig. 1.2 Conventional phases and tasks involved in biomedical text mining (Source: [44])

Text mining employs many computational technologies, such as machine learning, natural language processing, biostatistics, information technology, and pattern recognition, to find new exciting outcomes hidden in the unstructured biomedical text. There are many applications of cancer-related text mining [44], such as identifying malignant tumor-related biomedical mentions (genes, proteins, etc.), finding relationships among biomedical entities (protein–protein, gene–disease, etc.), extracting knowledge from text and generating hypotheses, and constructing or improving pathways.

The goal of text mining is to explore the implicit knowledge that remains hidden in unstructured text and present it in an explicit form. This generally has four phases:

1. Information retrieval
2. Information extraction
3. Knowledge discovery
4. Hypothesis generation

Information retrieval systems aim at getting required response to a given query; information extraction systems are used to extract predefined types of information such as relation extraction; knowledge discovery systems help us to extract novel knowledge from the text; hypothesis generation systems infer unknown biomedical facts based on the text. Thus, the general tasks of biomedical text mining include information retrieval, named entity recognition and relation extraction, knowledge discovery and hypothesis generation.

1.5 The Problem of Sentiment Analysis

In this section, we define an abstraction of the sentiment analysis problem [18]. This abstraction gives us a statement of the problem and enables us to see a rich set of interrelated subproblems. It is often said that if we cannot structure a problem, we probably do not understand the problem. The objective of the definitions thus far is to abstract a structure from the complex and intimidating unstructured natural language text. The structure serves as a common framework to unify various existing research directions and enables researchers to design more robust and accurate solution techniques by exploiting the interrelationships of the subproblems. From a practical application point of view, the definitions let practitioners see what subproblems need to be solved in building a sentiment analysis system, how the subproblems are related, and what output should be produced. Unlike factual information, sentiment and opinion have an important characteristic, namely, they are subjective. The subjectivity comes from many sources. First of all, different people may have different experiences and thus different opinions. For example, one person bought a camera of a particular brand and had a very good experience with it. She naturally has a positive opinion or sentiment about the camera. However, another person who also bought a camera of the same brand had some issues with it because he might just be unlucky and got a defective unit. He thus has a negative opinion. Second, different people may see the same thing in different ways because everything has two sides. For example, when the price of a stock is falling, one person may feel very sad because he bought the stock when the price was high, but another person may be very happy because it is an opportunity to short sell the stock to make good profits. Furthermore, different people may have different interests and/or different ideologies. Owing to such different subjective experiences, views, interests, and ideologies, it is important to examine a collection of opinions from many people rather than only one opinion from a single person, because such an opinion represents only the subjective view of that single person, which is usually not sufficient for action. With a large number of opinions, some form of summary [12] becomes necessary. Thus, the problem definition should also state what kind of summary may be desired. Along with the problem definitions, the chapter also discusses the important concepts of affect, emotion, and mood.

Conceptually, there is no fundamental difference between product reviews and other forms of opinion text, except some superficial differences and the degree of difficulty in dealing with them. For example, tweets are short (at most 140 characters) and informal, and often include Internet slang and emoticons which are explained in Sect. 2.5. Owing to the length limit, the authors are usually straight to the point. Thus, it is often easier to achieve a higher sentiment analysis accuracy for tweets. Reviews are also easier because they are highly focused with little irrelevant information. Forum discussions are perhaps the hardest to deal with because the users there can discuss anything and often are involved in interactive exchanges with one another. Different application domains also have different degrees of difficulty. Opinions about products and services are usually the easiest to deal with. Opinions about social and political issues are much harder because of complex topic and sentiment expressions, sarcasms [30], and ironies. These often need analysis at the pragmatics level, which can be difficult without sufficient background knowledge of the local social and political contexts. These explain why many commercial systems are able to perform sentiment analysis of opinions about products and services reasonably well but fare poorly on opinionated social and political texts. Sentiment analysis mainly studies opinions that express or imply positive or negative sentiment. We define the problem in this context. We use the term opinion as a broad concept that covers sentiment, evaluation, appraisal, or attitude and associated information such as opinion target and the person who holds the opinion, and we use the term sentiment to mean only the underlying positive or negative feeling implied by opinion. Owing to the need to analyze a large volume of opinions, in defining opinion, we consider two levels of abstraction: a single opinion and a set of opinions. According to [19];

An opinion is a quadruple,
(g,s, h, t),
where g is the sentiment target, s is the sentiment of the opinion about the target g, h is the opinion holder (the person or organization who holds the opinion), and t is the time when the opinion is expressed.

The four components here are essential. It is generally problematic if any of them is missing. For example, the time component is often very important in practice because an opinion 2 years ago is not the same as an opinion today. Not having an opinion holder is also problematic. For example, an opinion from a very important person (e.g., the prime minister of India) is probably more important than an opinion from an ordinary person.

1.5.1 Author and Reader Standpoint

We can look at an opinion from two perspectives [3], that of the author (opinion holder) who posts the opinion, and that of the reader who reads the opinion. Since opinions are subjective and depends on the context the reader and author take into account, naturally, the author and the reader may not see the same text in the same way. Let us use the following two example sentences to illustrate the point:
"Audi Q5 is too small for my family."
"Singapore's economy has gone up by +21.3% from 2006 to 2014."
Since the author or the opinion holder of the first sentence felt the Q5 is too small, a sentiment analysis system should output a negative opinion about the aspect: size of the car. However, this does not mean that the car is too small for everyone. A reader may actually feel the Q5's size big enough for his family and feel positive about

it. This causes a problem because if the system outputs only a negative opinion about size, the reader will not know whether it is too small or too large and then he/she would not see this positive aspect for him/her. Fortunately, this problem can be dealt with by mining and summarizing opinion reasons. Here 'too small' not only indicates a negative opinion about the size but also the reason for the negative opinion. With the reason, the reader can see a complete picture of the opinion. The second sentence represents a non-personal fact-implied opinion. Users can decide how to use the opinion based on their application needs. The final Sect. 1.6 introduces Deep Learning.

1.6 Deep Learning

The true challenge to AI proved to be solving the tasks that are easy for people to perform but hard for people to describe formally – problems that we solve intuitively, that feels automatic, like recognizing spoken words or faces in images. Hence, deep learning will allow computers to learn from experience and understand the world in terms of a hierarchy of concepts, with each concept defined in terms of its relation to simpler concepts. By gathering knowledge from experience, this approach avoids the need for human operators to formally specify all of the knowledge that the computer needs [16, 42]. The hierarchy of concepts will allow the computer to learn complicated concepts by building them out of simpler ones. If we draw a graph showing how these concepts are built on top of each other, the graph is deep, with multiple layers. For this reason, we call this approach to AI deep learning [13].

A major source of difficulty in many real-world AI applications is that many of the factors of variation influence every single piece of data we are able to observe. Of course, it can be very difficult to extract such high-level, abstract features from raw data. Many of these factors of variation, such as a speaker's accent, can be identified only using sophisticated, nearly human-level understanding of the data. When it is nearly as difficult to obtain a representation as to solve the original problem, representation learning does not, at first glance, seem to help us. Deep learning solves this central problem in representation learning by introducing representations that are expressed in terms of other, simpler representations. Deep learning allows the computer to build complex concepts out of simpler concepts. The Fig. 1.3 shows the deep learning architecture for textual data.

One of the questions which arise is how Deep Learning will help to solve such situations? The answer to that is:

1. It learns the right representation for the data provided either it could be image or a text
2. The depth allows the computer to learn a multi-step computer instruction.

In simpler words, each layer of the representation can be thought of as the state of the computer's memory after executing another set of instructions in parallel.

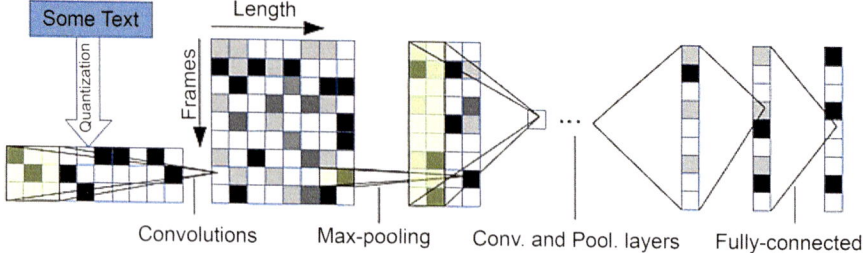

Fig. 1.3 Deep learning on textual data (Source: Authors)

Networks with greater depth can execute more instructions in sequence. In deep learning, the text is shown as a sequence of features instead of just a sequence of words or characters. The features could be tri-gram, bi-gram, and word2vec [24] to list a few. Deep learning methods are most effective when applied to large training sets, but in medicine, large datasets are not available. Few open-ended questions which need to be answered are:

1. Can deep networks be used effectively for medical tasks?
2. Is transfer learning from general imagery to the medical domain relevant?
3. Can we rely on learned features alone or may we combine them with handcrafted features for the task?

1.7   Organization of the Book

The rest of the book is organized as below:

1. Upcoming Chap. 2 discusses the Literature Survey associated with sentiment analysis and biomedical text mining. It dives into the importance of common-sense and covers its importance in human life and how it has the power to influence the world of AI.
2. The Chap. 3 introduces to SenticNet. SenticNet is about concept-level sentiment analysis, that is, performing tasks such as polarity detection and emotion recognition by leveraging on semantics and linguistics instead of solely relying on word co-occurrence frequencies.
3. The Chap. 4 introduces to Wordnet for Medical Events (WME). It discusses WME expansion and enriching WME with additional features. Finally, this chapter discusses combining computation creativity and machine learning.
4. The final Chap. 5 concludes the book with giving insights on the tools such as SenticNet and WME.

References

1. Boden, M.A.: The Creative Mind: Myths and Mechanisms. Basic Books, Inc., New York (1991)
2. Cambria, E.: Affective computing and sentiment analysis. IEEE Intell. Syst. **31**(2), 102–107 (2016)
3. Cambria, E., Das, D., Bandyopadhyay, S., Feraco, A.: A Practical Guide to Sentiment Analysis. Springer, Cham (2017)
4. Cambria, E., Livingstone, A., Hussain, A.: The hourglass of emotions. In: Esposito, A., Vinciarelli, A., Hoffmann, R., Muller, V. (eds.) Cognitive Behavioral Systems. Lecture Notes in Computer Science, vol. 7403, pp. 144–157. Springer, Berlin/Heidelberg (2012)
5. Cambria, E., Poria, S., Bajpai, R., Schuller, B.: Senticnet 4: a semantic resource for sentiment analysis based on conceptual primitives. In: Proceedings of COLING 2016, the 26th International Conference on Computational Linguistics: Technical Papers, pp. 2666–2677. The COLING 2016 Organizing Committee, Osaka (2016). http://aclweb.org/anthology/C16-1251
6. Cambria, E., Poria, S., Bisio, F., Bajpai, R., Chaturvedi, I.: The CLSA Model: A Novel Framework for Concept-Level Sentiment Analysis, pp. 3–22. Springer International Publishing, Cham (2015)
7. Cambria, E., Poria, S., Gelbukh, A., Thelwall, M.: Sentiment analysis is a big suitcase. IEEE Intell. Syst. **32**(6), 74–80 (2017)
8. Chaturvedi, I., Cambria, E., Vilares, D.: Lyapunov filtering of objectivity for Spanish sentiment model. In: IJCNN, Vancouver, pp. 4474–4481 (2016)
9. Chaturvedi, I., Ragusa, E., Gastaldo, P., Zunino, R., Cambria, E.: Bayesian network based extreme learning machine for subjectivity detection. J. Frankl. Inst. (2018). https://doi.org/10.1016/j.jfranklin.2017.06.007
10. Hogenboom, F., Frasincar, F., Kaymak, U., de Jong, F., Caron, E.: A survey of event extraction methods from text for decision support systems. Decis. Support Syst. **85**(C), 12–22 (2016). http://doi.org/10.1016/j.dss.2016.02.006
11. Hu, M., Liu, B.: Mining and summarizing customer reviews. In: Proceedings of the Tenth ACM SIGKDD International Conference on Knowledge Discovery and Data Mining, KDD'04, pp. 168–177. ACM, New York (2004). http://doi.org/10.1145/1014052.1014073
12. Hu, M., Liu, B.: Mining and summarizing customer reviews. In: Proceedings of the Tenth ACM SIGKDD International Conference on Knowledge Discovery and Data Mining, pp. 168–177. ACM (2004)
13. Ian, G., Yoshua, B., Aaron, C.: Deep learning. MIT Press (2016). http://www.deeplearningbook.org
14. Ikonomakis, M., Kotsiantis, S., Tampakas, V.: Text classification using machine learning techniques. WSEAS Trans. Comput. **4**(8), 966–974 (2005)
15. Koppel, M., Schler, J.: The importance of neutral examples for learning sentiment. Comput. Intell. **22**(2), 100–109 (2006). http://doi.org/10.1111/j.1467-8640.2006.00276.x
16. Li, Y., Pan, Q., Yang, T., Wang, S.H., Tang, J.L., Cambria, E.: Learning word representations for sentiment analysis. Cogn. Comput. **9**(6), 843–851 (2017)
17. Liu, B.: Sentiment analysis and subjectivity. In: Handbook of Natural Language Processing, 2nd edn. Taylor and Francis Group, Boca Raton (2010)
18. Liu, B.: Sentiment analysis and opinion mining. Synth. Lect. Hum. Lang. Technol. **5**(1), 1–167 (2012)
19. Liu, B.: Frontmatter. In: Sentiment Analysis: Mining Opinions, Sentiments, and Emotions, pp. i–iv. Cambridge University Press, Cambridge (2015)
20. Liu, B., Hu, M., Cheng, J.: Opinion observer: analyzing and comparing opinions on the web. In: Proceedings of the 14th International Conference on World Wide Web, WWW'05, pp. 342–351. ACM, New York (2005)

21. Ma, Y., Peng, H., Cambria, E.: Targeted aspect-based sentiment analysis via embedding commonsense knowledge into an attentive LSTM. In: Proceedings of AAAI (2018)

22. Manning, C.D., Schütze, H.: Foundations of Statistical Natural Language Processing. MIT Press, Cambridge (1999)

23. Mihalcea, R., Banea, C., Wiebe, J.: Learning multilingual subjective language via cross-lingual projections. In: ACL, Prague (2007)

24. Mikolov, T., Sutskever, I., Chen, K., Corrado, G.S., Dean, J.: Distributed representations of words and phrases and their compositionality. In: Advances in Neural Information Processing Systems, pp. 3111–3119 (2013)

25. Owyang, J.: The future of the social web: in five eras. Web 27 Apr 2009. www.web-strategist. com/blog/2009/04/27

26. Pang, B., Lee, L.: A sentimental education: sentiment analysis using subjectivity summarization based on minimum cuts. In: Proceedings of the 42Nd Annual Meeting on Association for Computational Linguistics, ACL '04. Association for Computational Linguistics, Stroudsburg (2004). http://doi.org/10.3115/1218955.1218990

27. Pang, B., Lee, L.: Seeing stars: exploiting class relationships for sentiment categorization with respect to rating scales. In: Proceedings of ACL, pp. 115–124 (2005)

28. Pang, B., Lee, L., Vaithyanathan, S.: Thumbs up?: sentiment classification using machine learning techniques. In: Proceedings of the ACL-02 Conference on Empirical Methods in Natural Language Processing – Volume 10, EMNLP '02, pp. 79–86. Association for Computational Linguistics, Stroudsburg (2002). http://doi.org/10.3115/1118693.1118704

29. Poria, S., Cambria, E., Bajpai, R., Hussain, A.: A review of affective computing: from unimodal analysis to multimodal fusion. Inf. Fusion **37**, 98–125 (2017)

30. Poria, S., Cambria, E., Hazarika, D., Vij, P.: A deeper look into sarcastic tweets using deep convolutional neural networks. In: COLING, pp. 1601–1612 (2016)

31. Poria, S., Chaturvedi, I., Cambria, E., Hussain, A.: Convolutional MKL based multimodal emotion recognition and sentiment analysis. In: ICDM, Barcelona, pp. 439–448 (2016)

32. Ribeiro, F.N., Araújo, M., Gonçalves, P., Benevenuto, F., Gonçalves, M.A.: A benchmark comparison of state-of-the-practice sentiment analysis methods. CoRR abs/1512.01818 (2015)

33. Russell, C.J., Bobko, P.: Moderated regression analysis and Likert scales: too coarse for comfort. J. Appl. Psychol. **77**(3), 336 (1992)

34. Snyder, B., Barzilay, R.: Multiple aspect ranking using the good grief algorithm. In: HLT/NAACL, Rochester (2007)

35. Socher, R., Perelygin, A., Wu, J.Y., Chuang, J., Manning, C.D., Ng, A.Y., Potts, C.: Recursive deep models for semantic compositionality over a sentiment treebank. In: EMNLP, pp. 1642–1654 (2013)

36. Su, F., Markert, K.: From words to senses: a case study of subjectivity recognition. In: Proceedings of the 22nd International Conference on Computational Linguistics – Volume 1, COLING'08, pp. 825–832. Association for Computational Linguistics, Stroudsburg (2008)

37. Taboada, M., Brooke, J., Tofiloski, M., Voll, K., Stede, M.: Lexicon-based methods for sentiment analysis. Comput. Linguist. **37**(2), 267–307 (2011)

38. Thelwall, M., Buckley, K., Paltoglou, G., Cai, D., Kappas, A.: Sentiment strength detection in short informal text. J. Am. Soc. Inf. Sci. Technol. **61**(12), 2544–2558 (2010). http://doi.org/10.1002/asi.21416

39. Titov, I., McDonald, R.: Modeling online reviews with multi-grain topic models. In: Proceedings of the 17th International Conference on World Wide Web, WWW'08, pp. 111–120. ACM, New York (2008). http://doi.org/10.1145/1367497.1367513

40. Turing, A.M.: Computing machinery and intelligence. Mind **59**(236), 433–460 (1950)

41. Turney, P.D.: Thumbs up or thumbs down? Semantic orientation applied to unsupervised classification of reviews. CoRR cs.LG/0212032 (2002)

42. Young, T., Hazarika, D., Poria, S., Cambria, E.: Recent trends in deep learning based natural language processing. IEEE Comput. Intell. Mag. (2018)

43. Zhai, Z., Liu, B., Xu, H., Jia, P.: Constrained LDA for grouping product features in opinion mining. In: Proceedings of the 15th Pacific-Asia Conference on Advances in Knowledge Discovery and Data Mining – Volume Part I, PAKDD'11, pp. 448–459. Springer, Berlin/Heidelberg (2011). http://dl.acm.org/citation.cfm?id=2017863.2017907

44. Zhu, F., Patumcharoenpol, P., Zhang, C., Yang, Y., Chan, J., Meechai, A., Vongsangnak, W., Shen, B.: Biomedical text mining and its applications in cancer research. J. Biomed. Inform. **46**(2), 200–211 (2013)

Chapter 2
Literature Survey

Abstract The best way to solve any problem is to reduce that problem to some problem whose solution is known. Similar approaches have been taken in the sentiment analysis as well. In this chapter, we discuss the importance of commonsense. This chapter will give an insight in the field of concept level sentiment analysis and Biomedical domain. It covers its importance in human life and how it has the power to influence the world of AI. The concept-level approach is the key to commonsense in AI. The following section introduces to different medical lexicons. Wordnet for Medical Events (WME) is the framework for medical concepts associated with real-world entities. Following medical lexicons, it discusses microtext analysis and levels of sentiment analysis. This chapter gives insights to Sentics. Sentics specifies the affective information associated with real-world entities, which holds the key for commonsense reasoning and decision-making.

Keywords Sentic computing • Affective computing • Sentiment analysis • Biomedical text mining • Natural language processing • Medical lexicons • Commonsense

Communication is one of the most important aspects of human life. Communication always gets associated with a cost in terms of energy and time, since information needs to be encoded and transmitted at the sender's end and decoded at the receiver's. On occasions, such factors can even make the difference between life and death. This is why people when communicating with each other, provide just the useful information and take the rest for granted. This '*taken for granted*' information is what is termed as 'commonsense' in human's way – obvious things people normally know and usually leave unstated while conversing. Commonsense is not the kind of knowledge we can find in Wikipedia, rather it implicitly exists in all the basic relationships among words, concepts, phrases, and thoughts that allow people to communicate with each other and face everyday life problems. It is a kind of knowledge that sounds obvious and natural to us but is actually ingenious and multifaceted. Humans leverage knowledge from the intuitions. Intuition can be explained as the process of making analogies between the current problem and the ones solved in the past to find a suitable solution. Marvin Minsky in [22] attributes this property to the so-called 'difference engines'. Affective computing

© Springer International Publishing AG 2017   21
R. Satapathy et al., *Sentiment Analysis in the Bio-Medical Domain*,
Socio-Affective Computing 7, https://doi.org/10.1007/978-3-319-68468-0_2

and sentiment analysis [2], hence, are key to the advancement of AI and all the research fields that stem from it. Sentiment-mining techniques can be exploited for the creation and automated upkeep of review and opinion aggregation websites, in which opinionated text and videos are continuously gathered from the Web and not restricted to just product reviews, but also to wider topics such as political issues and brand perception. Moreover, they find applications in various scenarios and companies, large and small, that include the analysis of emotions and sentiments as part of their mission.

2.1   Philosophy and Sentiments

Philosophical studies on emotions date back to ancient Greeks and Romans. Following the early Stoics, for example, Cicero enumerated and organized the emotions into four basic categories: *metus* (fear), *aegritudo* (pain), *libido* (lust), and *laetitia* (pleasure). Studies on the evolutionary theory of emotions, in turn, were initiated in the late nineteenth century by Darwin [8]. His thesis was that emotions evolved via natural selection and, therefore, have cross-culturally universal counterparts. In the early 1970s, Ekman found evidence that humans share six basic emotions: happiness, sadness, fear, anger, disgust, and surprise [10].

Few tentative efforts to detect non-basic affective states, such as fatigue, anxiety, satisfaction, confusion, or frustration, have been also made [6, 9, 17, 29, 32, 37] (Table 2.1). In 1980, Averill put forward the idea that emotions cannot be explained strictly on the basis of physiological or cognitive terms. Instead, he claimed that emotions are primarily social constructs; hence, a social level of analysis is necessary to truly understand the nature of emotion [1].

Table 2.1 Some existing definition of basic emotions. The most widely adopted model for affect recognition is Ekman's, although is one of the poorest in terms of number of emotions (Source: [3])

Author	#Emotions	Basic emotions
Ekman	6	Anger, disgust, fear, joy, sadness, surprise
Parrot	6	Anger, fear, joy, love, sadness, surprise
Frijda	6	Desire, happiness, interest, surprise, wonder, sorrow
Plutchik	8	Acceptance, anger, anticipation, disgust, joy, fear, sadness, surprise
Tomkins	9	Desire, happiness, interest, surprise, wonder, sorrow
Matsumoto	22	Joy, anticipation, anger, disgust, sadness, surprise, fear, acceptance, shy, pride, appreciate, calmness, admire, contempt, love, happiness, exciting, regret, ease, discomfort, respect, like

The relationship between emotion and language (and the fact that the language of emotion is considered a vital part of the experience of emotion) has been used by social constructivists and anthropologists to question the universality of Ekman's studies, arguably because the language labels he used to code emotions are somewhat US-centric. In addition, other cultures might have labels that cannot be literally translated into English (e.g., some languages do not have a word for fear [36]). For their deep connection with language and for the limitedness of the emotional labels used, all such categorical approaches usually fail to describe the complex range of emotions that can occur in daily communication. The dimensional approach [26], in turn, represents emotions as coordinates in a multi-dimensional space.

For both theoretical and practical reasons, an increasing number of researchers like to define emotions according to two or more dimensions. An early example is Russell's circumplex model [35], which uses the dimensions of arousal and valence to plot 150 affective labels. Similarly, Whissell considers emotions as a continuous 2D space whose dimensions are evaluation and activation [43]. The evaluation dimension measures how a human feels, from positive to negative. The activation dimension measures whether humans are more or less likely to take some action under the emotional state, from active to passive. In her study, Whissell assigns a pair of values ⟨activation, evaluation⟩ to each of the approximately 9,000 words with affective connotations that make up her Dictionary of Affect in Language.

Another bi-dimensional model is Plutchik's wheel of emotions, which offers an integrative theory based on evolutionary principles [30]. Following Darwin's thought, the functionalist approach to emotions holds that emotions have evolved for a particular function, such as to keep the subject safe [13, 14]. Emotions are adaptive as they have a complexity born of a long evolutionary history and, although we conceive emotions as feeling states, Plutchik says the feeling state is part of a process involving both cognition and behavior and containing several feedback loops. In 1980, he created a wheel of emotions, which consisted of eight basic emotions and eight advanced emotions each composed of two basic ones.

Besides bi-dimensional approaches, a commonly used set for emotion dimension is the <arousal, valence, dominance> set, which is known in the literature also by different names, including <evaluation, activation, power> and <pleasure, arousal, dominance> [21]. Recent evidence suggests there should be a fourth dimension: Fontaine et al. reported consistent results from various cultures where a set of four dimensions is found in user studies, namely <valence, potency, arousal, unpredictability> [12]. Dimensional representations of affect are attractive mainly because they provide a way of describing emotional states that are more tractable than using words. This is of particular importance when dealing with naturalistic data, where a wide range of emotional states occurs. Similarly, they are much more able to deal with non-discrete emotions and variations in emotional states over time [7], since in such cases changing from one universal emotion label to another would not make much sense in real life scenarios. Dimensional approaches, however, have a few limitations. Although the dimensional space allows comparing affect words according to their reciprocal distance, it usually does not allow making operations between these, e.g., for studying compound emotions. Most dimensional representations, moreover, do not model the fact that two or more emotions may be experienced at the same time. Eventually, all such approaches work at the word-level, which makes them unable to grasp the affective valence of multiple-word concepts (Fig. 2.1).

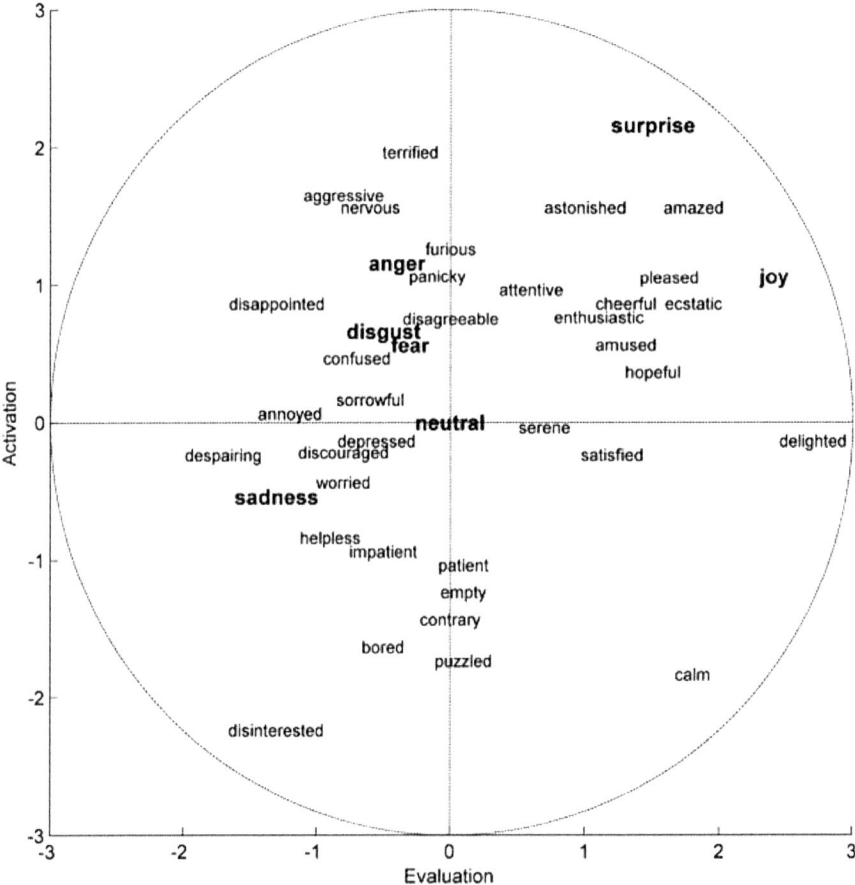

Fig. 2.1 Whissell's model is a bi-dimensional representation of emotions, in which words from the Dictionary of Affect in Language are displayed. The diagram shows the position of some of these words in the < activation, evaluation > space (Source: Hour Glass Model [4])

2.2 Importance of Commonsense

Commonsense is the holistic knowledge (usually acquired in early stages of our lives) concerning all the social, political, economic, and environmental aspects of the society we live in. Computers can only do logical things, but the meaning is an intuitive process – it cannot be simply reduced to zeros and ones. We will need to transmit to computers our commonsense knowledge of the world as there may actually not be enough capable human workers left to perform the necessary tasks for our rapidly ageing population. To deal with this emerging AI emergency,[1] we will be required to endow computers and machines with physical knowledge of how objects behave, social knowledge of how people interact, sensory knowledge of how things look and taste, psychological knowledge about the way people think, and so on. However, having a simple database of millions of commonsense facts will not be enough: we will also have to teach computers how to handle and make sense of this knowledge, retrieve it when necessary, and contextually learn from experience – in a word, we will have to give them the capacity for commonsense reasoning.

Natural language processing research has been interspersed with word-level approaches. The reason being at first glance, the most basic unit of the linguistic structure appears to be a word. However, single-word expressions, are just a subset of concepts. Concepts are multi-word expressions that express specific semantics and sentics, that is, "the denotative and connotative information commonly associated with real-world objects, actions, events, and people". Sentics [3], in particular, specifies the affective information associated with such real-world entities, which is key for commonsense reasoning and decision-making. Semantics and Sentics both include commonsense knowledge (which we humans generally gain during the initial years of our life) and common knowledge (which we continue to learn throughout our life) in a reusable knowledge base (KB) for machines. Common knowledge includes general knowledge about the world, e.g., "cricket is a type of sports", while commonsense knowledge consists of obvious or widely accepted things, which people normally know about the world but which are usually left unstated in discourse, e.g., that "things fall downwards (and not upwards)" and "people smile when they are happy". The difference between common knowledge and commonsense knowledge can be expressed as the difference between knowing the name of an object and understanding the same object's purpose. For example, you can know the name of all the different kinds or brands of 'cars', but not its purpose nor the method of usage. In other words, a 'car' in Fig. 2.2 is not a car unless we know how to drive it.

---

[1]http://mitworld.mit.edu/video/484

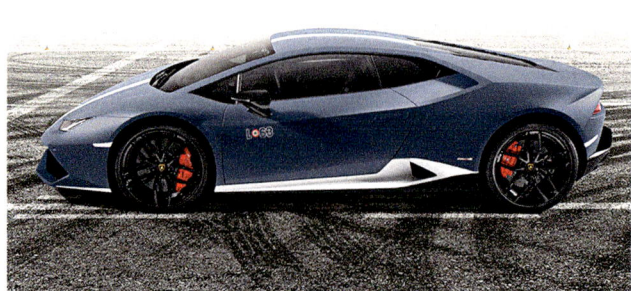

Fig. 2.2 Lamborghini is not a car unless you know how to ride it

2.3 Medical Lexicons

In the domain of clinical text processing, sense-based information extraction is considered as a challenging task due to the unstructured nature of the corpus. The difficulty in preparing structured corpora for the clinical domain is because of the little/no involvement of the domain experts. A term is a name used in a specific domain, and a terminology is a collection of terms. Terms abound in the Biomedical text, where they constitute important building blocks. Some examples of terms are the names of cell types, proteins, medical devices, diseases, symptoms, gene mutations, chemical names, and protein domains [33].

2.3.1 Why a Medical Lexicon

The biomedical text is not a homogeneous realm. Medical records are written differently from scientific articles, sequence annotations, or public health guidelines. Moreover, local dialects are not uncommon. For example, medical centers and laboratories use different words with the same meaning. This variability means, in practice, that text mining applications are tailored to specific types of text. A consumer health information system must be able to comprehend both experts and non-experts medical vocabulary and to map between the two.

2.3.1.1 Mismatches in Doctor-Patient Communication

This subsection tries to understand why is there a need of a standard lexicon. It depicts the differences between the patients and doctors communication with an example. The skills of a physician in general practice comprise the ability to acquire relevant and reliable information through communication with patients through the use of non-expert language and to convey diagnostic and therapeutic information in ways tailored to the individual patient. Since, physicians, too, are a member of the wider community of non-experts, and continues to use the non-expert language for everyday purposes, one might assume that there are no difficulties in principle keeping him/her from being able to formulate medical knowledge in a vocabulary that the patient can understand. As [38] and [40] have shown, however, there are limits to this competence. The former examines dialogue between physicians and patients in the form of question-answer pairs, focusing especially on the relations documented in the UMLS Semantic Network. Only about 30% of the relations used by professionals in their answers directly match the relations used by consumers in formulating their questions. An example of one such famous question-answer pair taken from [38] is as follows:

Question Text: My seven-year-old son developed a rash today that I believe to be chickenpox. My concern is that a friend of mine had her 10-day-old baby at my home last evening before we were aware of the illness. My son had no contact with the infant, as he was in bed during the visit, but I have read that chickenpox is contagious up to 2 days prior to the actual rash. Is there cause for concern at this point?

Answer Text:

1. Chickenpox is the common name for varicella infection.
2. You are correct in that a person with chickenpox can be contagious for 48 h before the first vesicle is seen.
3. The fact that your son did not come in close contact with the infant means he most likely did not transmit the virus.
4. Of concern, though, is the fact that newborns are at higher risk of complications of varicella, including pneumonia.
5. There is a very effective means to prevent infection after exposure. A form of an antibody to varicella called varicella-zoster immune globulin (VZIG) can be given up to 48 h after exposure and still prevent disease. Such examples illustrate also that there are lexically rooted mismatches in communication (which may in part reflect legal and ethical considerations) between experts and non-experts. Professionals often do not reuse the concepts and relations made explicit in the questions put to them by consumers. In our example, the questioner requests a yes/no-judgment on the possibility of contagion in a 10-day-old baby. Physicians expand the range of concepts and relations addressed (for example, through discussion of issues of prevention, etc.,). Hence, the medical lexicons help to map generic medical information which non-experts are able to understand and preserve the technicalities as the same time.

2.3.1.2   Non-expert Language in Online Communication

Understanding patients require both explicit medical knowledge and also tacit linguistic competence that is dispersed across large numbers of more or less isolated practitioners. This is not a problem so long as this knowledge is to be applied locally, in face-to-face communication with patients. However, as a result of recent developments in technology, including telemedicine and Internet-based medical query systems, we now face a situation where such dispersed, practical (human) knowledge does not suffice. Online communication includes conversing in microtexts which are explained in detail in Sect. 2.5. In the context of Bio-medical corpora, the medical terms (events) and their related information extraction can help to develop an annotation system, which is essential for representing the structured corpus. Biomedical information extraction research is challenging due to lack of complete structured corpus on the contrary to a huge amount of semi-structured and unstructured medical corpora. In [42], UzZaman generates an event and temporal expression extraction from raw text. The researchers have introduced the domain- specific lexicons with preserving the features such as polarity score, semantics, and sentiment (sense) for medical concepts to build information extraction systems considering annotation and relation identification from unstructured medical corpora [42]. To this end, the standard tool as GENIA tagger [25] and the lexicons MEN (Medical WordNet) [39] and WME (WordNet of Medical Event) [24] have been constructed. MEN lexicon has been built with two sub-networks, namely Medical FactNet (MFN) and Medical BeliefNet (MBN), to evaluate consumer health reports [39]. Wordnet of Medical Events (WME) [23] started with the aim of having a medical lexicon. As there is no state of the art medical lexicon, it is difficult to say whether the one created is the best and even more difficult to compare the results. For that, we have made efforts to expand the lexicon in terms of features as well as concepts. That is, the most important information of medical word is associated with the word/concept itself and can be stored in a lexicon. However, contextual information is also important, and this relationship can be modeled only after a manually or automated training corpus is built.

2.4   Lexicons in BioNLP Domain

This section lists the lexicons in BioNLP domain. It includes MFN, MWN, MBN, and WME.

2.4.1   MFN

MFN consists of those sentences in the corpus which receives high marks for correctness on being assessed by medical experts. MFN is thus designed to constitute a representative fraction of the true beliefs about medical phenomena which are intelligible to non-expert English-speakers. The ultimate goal of our work on MFN is to document the entirety of the medical knowledge that is capable of being understood by average adult consumers of healthcare services in the United States today who have no special knowledge of medical phenomena.

2.4.2 MWN

MWN is based on WordNet which is a large electronic lexical database of English. Wordnet was originally conceived as a full-scale model of human semantic organization, where words and their meanings are related to one another via semantic and lexical relations.The building block of WordNet is a synonym set, or synset, consisting of all the words that can be substituted for one another in given types of sentential contexts without change of truth value in the sentences involved. Not all the members of a given synset will be interchangeable in all contexts. For example, the synsets "car, automobile" and "vehicle" are connected to each other through the hypernymy/hyponymy relation; "wheel" and "car" are linked via the meronymy/holonymy relation. In principle, WordNet's structure should ensure that all hyponyms (types) of "car" are also hyponyms of "vehicle" (and that all hyponyms of "car" refer to objects having referents of "wheel" as parts). While WordNet's current version has broad medical context coverage, it manifests a number of defects, which reflect both the lack of domain expertise on the part of the responsible lexicographers and also the fact that WordNet was not built for domain-specific applications.

2.4.3 MBN

MBN consists of those sentences in the corpus which receive high marks for assent. MBN is thus designed to constitute a representative fraction of the beliefs about medical phenomena (both true and false) distributed through the population of English speakers. Compiling MFN and MBN in tandem will allow systematic assessment of the disparity between lay beliefs and vocabulary as concerns medical phenomena and the corresponding expert medical knowledge.

2.4.4 WME

Author's envisage the WME lexicon [24] being used in the fields of medical education and medical literacy to evaluate the reliability of the medical knowledge of different experts and non-expert communities. On the basis of structured data pertaining to the sources of entries in WME, it will be possible to keep track of specific kinds of diseases and symptoms as originating in specific populations of informants. This may prove a valuable source of information in targeting particular groups for specific types of remedial medical education. WME will help in automating the process of symptom extraction from the text and providing remedies specific to the population. For ex: people from Europe and India even though showing from similar diseases may need to be handled with different drugs.

2.4.4.1   WME 1.0

The seed list of WME resource has been prepared from the trial and training datasets of the SemEval-2015 Task-6.[2] The conventional WordNet and English medical dictionary were applied on the seed list for developing the initial WME resource. Primarily, the resource extracted 2479 numbers of medical events along with their attributes such as type, span context, sense (positive or negative) from the provided datasets. Several polarity lexicons like SentiWordNet, Taboada's adjective list were used for identifying the appropriate gloss of the medical events from file context, WordNet definition and dictionary gloss of the medical events.

2.4.4.2   WME2.0

The new seed list was prepared from a medical domain on the web. New medical words were added to its previous list after the removal of noise (like non-medical terms). Further, it was expanded with the addition of new features. The inclusion of semantic and knowledge-based features is crucial for preparing the expanded version of existing resource, WME 1.0 which we will call as WME2.0. The semantic, polarity, sense and affinity features have been employed; as these features help to identify and extract the medical events from the clinical corpus. The updated lexicon has been converted to a **diseases x symptom** matrix from which a lot of new information like similar disease/symptom, new disease/symptom convergence has been done. This information could leverage information for the new and unknown diseases. There could be a hidden disease due to an addition or removal of a particular symptom. Further evaluation has been shown in Chap. 4.

2.5   Microtext Analysis

Microtexts are short snippets of text found in many modes of communication: microblogs (e.g., Twitter, Reddit), Short Message Streams (SMS), chat (e.g., instant messaging, Internet Relay Chat), and transcribed conversations (e.g., FBI hostage

---

[2]http://alt.qcri.org/semeval2015/task6/

negotiations). Microtext often has the characteristics of informality, brevity, varied grammar, frequent misspellings (both accidental and purposeful), and usage of abbreviations, acronyms, and emoticons. With more conversational forms of microtext such as multi-participant chat, there are also entangled conversation threads. These characteristics create many difficulties for analyzing and understanding microtext, often causing traditional NLP techniques to fail. Research on microtext is becoming increasingly necessary given the explosion of online microtext language. Yet, very few suitable tools have been developed for analyzing it. Also, there are few sufficiently-large publicly-available data sets (such as the Twitter corpus[3]). Currently, most NLP tools are designed to deal with grammatical, properly spelled and punctuated language corpora. However, the reality is that a vast portion of online data does not conform to the canons of standard grammar and spelling. For example, "M feelin vry hppy 2de" is one of the many tweets in microtext. In this example, the sentence needs to be normalized to "I am feeling very happy today". Hence, there is a growing need for specialized tools that tolerate noisy and fragmented microtext. The first step in tackling this challenge is to realize that, while the number of different spelling variations may be massive, they follow a small number of simple basic strategies as in [11]:

1. **Abbreviation**: The user may delete letters (typically vowels) from the word. For example, in the Twitter corpus studied in [11], the word "together" was found sometimes rendered as "tgthr".
2. **Phonetic substitution**: The user may substitute letters for other symbols that sound the same. This is typically done by using homophonic numbers, such as "2" for "to" in "2gether".
3. **Graphemic substitution**: The user might substitute a letter for a symbol that looks the same. A common example is switching a letter "o" for the number "0", such as in "t0gether".
4. **Stylistic variation**: The user misspells the word to make it look more like its phonetic pronunciation (or sometimes specifically the user's pronunciation).

The variations of normal texts are called out-of-vocabulary and are required to be converted to normal texts which are called in-vocabulary texts. Bringing together researchers from various fields to discuss microtext analysis will pave the way towards bringing the NLP methods, tools, and corpora in line with the current needs of the NLP community in academia, industry, and government. Application of microtext analysis varies from sentiment analysis of chats and tweets to stopping online piracy. One of the real life example is the name of the movie "Snowden" written as "Sn0wd3n" and gets uploaded to the torrent, thereby making it difficult to track [18]. The term microtext was proposed by US Navy researchers [34] to describe a type of written text document that has three characteristics:

---

[3]https://dev.twitter.com/overview/api

1. It is very short, typically one or two sentences, and possibly as little as a single word;
2. It is written in an informal manner and unedited for quality, and thus may use loose grammar, a conversational tone, vocabulary errors, and uncommon abbreviations and acronyms; and
3. It is semi-structured in the NLP sense, in that it includes some metadata such as a time stamp, an author, or the name of a field it was entered into.

Microtexts have become omnipresent in today's world: they are notably found everywhere from online chat discussions, online forum posts, user comments posted on online resources such as videos, pictures and news stories, Facebook news feeds and Twitter updates, internet search queries, to phone text messaging (SMS). The microtext processing refers to the branch of NLP that focuses on handling informal texts. The processing tasks found within this branch overlaps greatly with those in more traditional text processing areas, which includes summarization, sentiment analysis, topic detection and classification, question-answering, and information extraction. The importance of microtext processing cannot be overstated. With the passage of everyday, billions of new microtexts are published. Furthermore, these microtexts are rich in information, not only in their textual content but also in their associated metadata. This information is of value for NLP research, as well as for practical data mining application for social networking sites, web search engines, telecommunication companies, marketing firms, news sites, and many others. The types and features of microtexts are directly dependent on the nature of the technological support that makes them possible. The birth of microtext is a direct result of the development in telecommunication technology and Internet. Although microtexts were used as early as the 1980s, it was in the mid-1990s that their popularity expanded, as a result of the commercialization of the GSM mobile phone network with SMS support starting from 1993, and the release of numerous user-friendly IRC and IM software post 1995. The scientific community quickly took notice of these emerging text corpora, and began using them in research projects. We can initially differentiate two branches of research: on the linguistics side scientists performed research about microtext, while on the NLP side they performed research using microtext. Some of the unique features of microtext, which are highlighted in Ellens definition [34], were immediately obvious to linguists. In fact, as early as 1991, researchers studying what they called interactive written discourse on TELENET (a precursor of the Internet) had noticed that the messages exchanged there were different from the standard English and that the users omitted pronouns, articles and copulas, used uncommon abbreviations, and featured incorrect capital-ization. These researchers were among the first to note that these e-messages, as they were called, should not be categorized as either written or spoken English but represented a new form of the language. Over the following decades, other linguists who studied chat messaging, SMS, and IM, echoed and expanded on these observations. New linguistic features, such as the use of phonetic substitutions ('u' for 'you', 'r' for 'are') [28] and the omission of punctuation [20], were catalogued. Over time, the full social impact became appreciated: this was not a local trend among online friends but a socially prevalent [28] and international phenomenon as in [20]. However, referring to the definition in [34], these linguists overlooked the existence of metadata associated with the messages. On the NLP side, the opposite approach was initially prevalent. Researchers sought to fit microtext corpora into the existing theoretical framework they were familiar with and use tried-and-true NLP methodologies. This typically meant preprocessing a corpus to make it more similar to a regular English text corpus. For example, when researchers in [19] wanted to implement a chat room topic detection method, they stripped all metadata from the chat messages and merged them all together into a single string, then arbitrarily split that string into what they called pseudo-documents. This pre-processing allowed them to apply classical NLP methods to build document vectors for each pseudo-document and classify them. It wasn't before 2002 that NLP researchers began noting that chat conversations differ in significant ways from regular text. From there, they began to rediscover the linguistic features that linguists had been cataloguing for over a decade, and additionally noted that the surrounding metadata could be mined for information as well. The three key features of the texts are that, they are short, written informally, and include metadata – were observed together for the first time, but specifically as important distinctive attributes of IM compared to regular text. It would not until [34] suggested that microtext was a separate class of text which encompassed IRC, IM, SMS, social network updates and more, and which was functionally defined by these three attributes. By that time, research about microtext was becoming common in the NLP branch of research as well, with new projects exploiting the unique features of microtext. Thus, in a sense, the NLP branch combined with and enriched the linguistic branch, and together they gave us this new field of microtext processing. Text Message Normalization One of the fundamental characteristics of microtext is a highly relaxed spelling and a reliance on uncommon abbreviations and acronyms. This causes problems when we try to apply traditional NLP tools and techniques (such as Information extraction, automated summarization, or text-to-speech) that have been developed for conventional English text. It could be thought that a simple find-and-replace preprocessing on the microtext would solve that problem. However, the sheer diversity of spelling variations makes this solution impractical; Moreover, new spelling variations are created constantly, both voluntarily and accidentally. The challenge of developing algorithms to correct the out-of-vocabulary found in microtexts is known as Text Message Normalization (TMN).

2.6 Different Levels of Sentiment Analysis

This section introduces to the main research problems based on the level of granularities in the field of sentiment analysis. Level of granularity is decided by the application purpose. For example, if sentiment analysis is to be done on a blog or news article then we need document level granularity. In general, sentiment analysis has been investigated mainly at four levels:

1. *Document level:* The task at this level is to classify whether a whole opinion document expresses a positive or negative sentiment [27, 41]. For example, given a product review, the system determines whether the review expresses an overall positive or negative opinion about the product. This task is commonly known as document-level sentiment classification. This level of analysis assumes that each document expresses opinions on a single entity (e.g., a single product). Thus, it is not applicable to documents which evaluate or compare multiple entities.

2. *Sentence level:* The task at this level goes to the sentences and determines whether each sentence expressed a positive, negative, or neutral opinion. Neutral usually means no opinion. This level of analysis is closely related to subjectivity classification [44], which distinguishes sentences otherwise called as objective sentences that express factual information from the subjective sentences that express subjective views and opinions. However, we should note that subjectivity is not equivalent to sentiment as many objective sentences can imply opinions, e.g., "We bought the car last month and the windshield wiper has fallen off". Researchers have also analyzed clauses [45], but the clause level is still not enough, e.g., "Apple is doing very well in this lousy economy".

3. *Entity and Aspect level:* Both the document level and the sentence level analyses do not discover what exactly people liked and did not like. Aspect level performs a finer grained analysis. Aspect level was earlier called feature level (feature-based opinion mining and summarization) [15]. Instead of looking at language constructs in documents, paragraphs, sentences, clauses or phrases, aspect level directly looks at the opinion itself. It is based on the idea that an opinion consists of a sentiment (a positive or a negative) and a target (of opinion). An opinion without its target being identified is of limited use. Realizing the importance of opinion targets also helps us understand the sentiment analysis problem better. For example, although the sentence "although the service is not that great, I still love this restaurant" clearly has a positive tone, we cannot say that this sentence is entirely positive. In fact, the sentence is positive about the restaurant (emphasized) but negative about its service (not emphasized). In many applications, opinion targets are described by entities and/or their different aspects. Thus, the goal of this level of analysis is to discover sentiments on entities and/or their aspects. For example, the sentence "The iPhone's call quality is good, but its battery life is short" evaluates two aspects, "call quality" and "battery life", of iPhone which is an entity. The sentiment on iPhone's call quality is positive, but the sentiment on its battery life is negative. The call quality and battery life of iPhone are the opinion targets. Based on this level of analysis, a structured summary of opinions about entities and their aspects can be produced, which turns unstructured text to structured data and can be used for all kinds of qualitative and quantitative analyses. Both the document level and sentence level classifications are already highly challenging. The aspect-level is even more difficult.

4. *Concept Level:* Concept-level sentiment analysis [3] is a natural language processing (NLP) task that has recently raised growing interest both within the scientific community, leading to many exciting open challenges, as well as in the

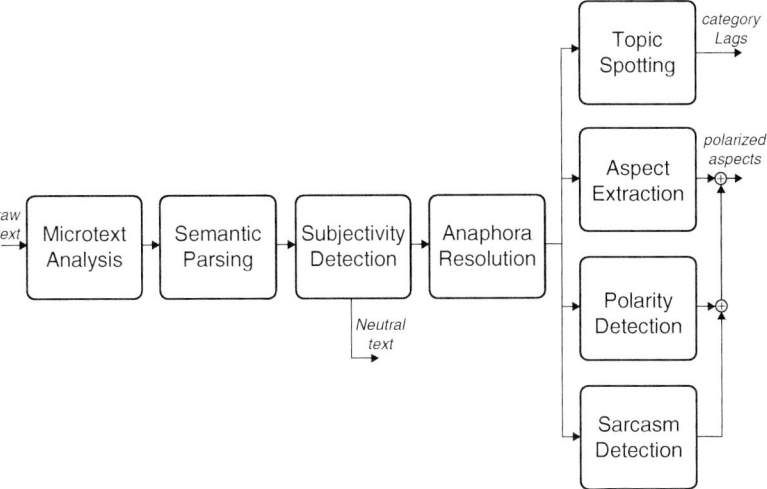

Fig. 2.3 Concept level sentiment analysis (Source: [5])

business world, due to the remarkable benefits to be had from financial market prediction. The potential applications of concept-level sentiment analysis, in fact, are countless and span interdisciplinary areas such as political forecasting, brand positioning, and human-robot interaction. CLSA model as a reference framework for researchers willing to take a more holistic and semantic-aware approach to sentiment analysis, which also applies to the multimodal realm [31] (Fig. 2.3). The main contributions of the proposed model are as follows:

(a) it promotes the analysis of opinionated text at concept, rather than word-level, and

(b) it takes into account all the NLP tasks necessary for extracting opinionated information from text

To make things even more interesting and challenging, there are two types of opinions, i.e.,

1. regular opinions, and;
2. comparative opinions [16]

A regular opinion expresses a sentiment only on a particular entity or an aspect of the entity, e.g., "Milo tastes very good," which expresses a positive sentiment on the aspect taste of Milo. A comparative opinion compares multiple entities based on some of their shared aspects, e.g., "Milo tastes better than Bournvita," which compares Milo and Bournvita based on their tastes (an aspect) and expresses a preference for Milo by an individual.

2.7   Sentic Patterns

This section introduces how SenticNet can be used for the sentiment analysis
task of polarity detection (Fig. 2.4). In particular, a semantic parser is firstly used
to deconstruct natural language text into concepts (Sect. 3.4). Secondly, linguistic
patterns are used in concomitance with SenticNet to infer polarity from sentences.
If no match is found in SenticNet or in the linguistic patterns, machine learning is
used (Sect. 3.5). Finally, it discusses a comparative evaluation of the framework with
respect to the state of the art in polarity detection from the text. The next chapter
introduces to SenticNet in detail.

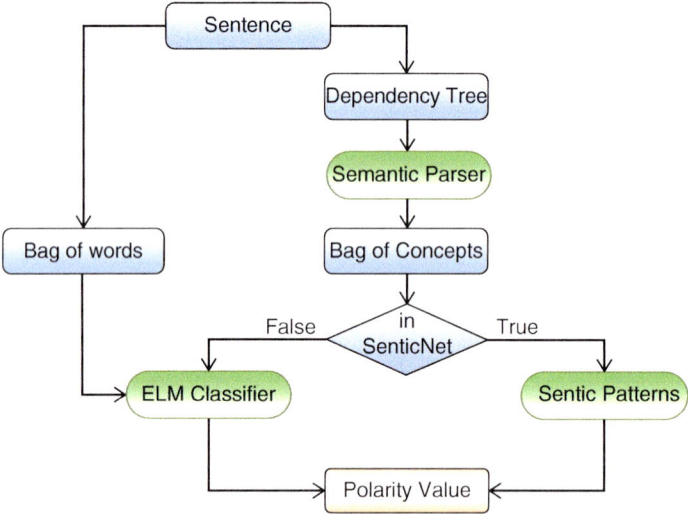

Fig. 2.4 Flowchart of the sentence-level polarity detection framework. The text is first decom-
posed into concepts. If these are found in SenticNet, sentic patterns are applied. If none of the
concepts are available in SenticNet, the ELM classifier is employed (Source: Sentic computing [3])

References

1. Averill, J.: A constructivist view of emotion. In: Plutchik, R., Kellerman, H. (eds.) Emotion:
   Theory, Research and Experience, pp. 305–339. Academic Press, New York (1980)
2. Cambria, E.: Affective computing and sentiment analysis. IEEE Intell. Syst. **31**(2), 102–107
   (2016)
3. Cambria, E., Hussain, A.: Sentic Computing: A Common-Sense-Based Framework for
   Concept-Level Sentiment Analysis. Springer, Cham (2015)
4. Cambria, E., Livingstone, A., Hussain, A.: The hourglass of emotions. In: Esposito, A.,
   Vinciarelli, A., Hoffmann, R., Muller, V. (eds.) Cognitive Behavioral Systems. Lecture Notes
   in Computer Science, vol. 7403, pp. 144–157. Springer, Berlin/Heidelberg (2012)

5. Cambria, E., Poria, S., Bisio, F., Bajpai, R., Chaturvedi, I.: The CLSA Model: A Novel Framework for Concept-Level Sentiment Analysis, pp. 3–22. Springer International Publishing, Cham (2015)

6. Castellano, G., Kessous, L., Caridakis, G.: Multimodal emotion recognition from expressive faces, body gestures and speech. In: Doctoral Consortium of ACII, Lisbon (2007)

7. Cochrane, T.: Eight dimensions for the emotions. Soc. Sci. Inf. **48**(3), 379–420 (2009)

8. Darwin, C.: The Expression of the Emotions in Man and Animals. John Murray, London (1872)

9. Douglas-Cowie, E.: Humaine deliverable D5g: mid term report on database exemplar progress. Tech. rep., Information Society Technologies (2006)

10. Ekman, P., Dalgleish, T., Power, M.: Handbook of Cognition and Emotion. Wiley, Chichester (1999)

11. Fei, L., Fuliang, W., Bingqing, W., Yang, L.: Insertion, deletion, or substitution? Normalizing text messages without pre-categorization nor supervision (2011)

12. Fontaine, J., Scherer, K., Roesch, E., Ellsworth, P.: The world of emotions is not two-dimensional. Psycholog. Sci. **18**(12), 1050–1057 (2007)

13. Freitas, A., Castro, E.: Facial expression: the effect of the smile in the treatment of depression. empirical study with Portuguese subjects. In: Emotional Expression: The Brain and The Face, pp. 127–140. University Fernando Pessoa Press (2009)

14. Frijda, N.H.: The laws of emotions. Am. Psychol. **43**(5), 349 (1988)

15. Hu, M., Liu, B.: Mining and summarizing customer reviews. In: Proceedings of the Tenth ACM SIGKDD International Conference on Knowledge Discovery and Data Mining, pp. 168–177. ACM (2004)

16. Jindal, N., Liu, B.: Identifying comparative sentences in text documents. In: Proceedings of the 29th Annual International ACM SIGIR Conference on Research and Development in Information Retrieval, SIGIR'06, pp. 244–251. ACM, New York (2006). http://doi.org/10.1145/1148170.1148215

17. Kapoor, A., Burleson, W., Picard, R.: Automatic prediction of frustration. Int. J. Hum.-Comput. Stud. **65**, 724–736 (2007)

18. Khoury, R., Khoury, R., Hamou-Lhadj, A.: Microtext Processing. Springer, New York (2014)

19. Kolenda, T., Hansen, L.K., Larsen, J.: Signal detection using ICA: application to chat room topic spotting, pp. 540–545 (2001)

20. Ling, R., Baron, N.S.: Text messaging and IM. J. Lang. Soc. Psychol. **26**(3), 291–298 (2007). http://doi.org/10.1177/0261927X06303480

21. Mehrabian, A.: Pleasure-arousal-dominance: a general framework for describing and measuring individual differences in temperament. Curr. Psychol. **14**(4), 261–292 (1996)

22. Minsky, M.: The Society of Mind. Simon and Schuster, New York (1986)

23. Mondal, A., Chaturvedi, I., Das, D., Bajpai, R., Bandyopadhyay, S.: Lexical resource for medical events: a polarity based approach. In: ICDM Workshops, pp. 1302–1309. IEEE (2015)

24. Mondal, A., Das, D., Cambria, E., Bandyopadhyay, S.: WME: sense, polarity and affinity based concept resource for medical events. In: Proceedings of the Eighth Global WordNet Conference, pp. 242–246 (2016)

25. Ohta, T., Tateisi, Y., Kim, J.D.: The GENIA corpus: an annotated research abstract corpus in molecular biology domain. In: Proceedings of the Second International Conference on Human Language Technology Research, HLT'02, pp. 82–86. Morgan Kaufmann Publishers Inc., San Francisco (2002). http://dl.acm.org/citation.cfm?id=1289189.1289260

26. Osgood, C., Suci, G., Tannenbaum, P.: The Measurement of Meaning. University of Illinois Press, Urbana (1957)

27. Pang, B., Lee, L., Vaithyanathan, S.: Thumbs up?: sentiment classification using machine learning techniques. In: Proceedings of the ACL-02 Conference on Empirical Methods in Natural Language Processing – Volume 10, EMNLP '02, pp. 79–86. Association for Computational Linguistics, Stroudsburg (2002). http://doi.org/10.3115/1118693.1118704

28. Paolillo, J.C.: Formalizing formality: an analysis of register variation in Sinhala. J. Linguist. **36**(2), 215–259 (2000). http://www.jstor.org/stable/4176592
29. Parrott, W.: Emotions in Social Psychology. Psychology Press, Philadelphia (2001)
30. Plutchik, R.: The nature of emotions. Am. Sci. **89**(4), 344–350 (2001)
31. Poria, S., Chaturvedi, I., Cambria, E., Hussain, A.: Convolutional MKL based multimodal emotion recognition and sentiment analysis. In: ICDM, Barcelona, pp. 439–448 (2016)
32. Prinz, J.: Gut Reactions: A Perceptual Theory of Emotion. Oxford University Press, Oxford (2004)
33. Rodriguez-Esteban, R.: Biomedical text mining and its applications. PLoS Comput. Biol. **5**(12), e1000597 (2009)
34. Rosa, K.D., Ellen, J.: Text classification methodologies applied to micro-text in military chat. In: Proceedings of the 2009 International Conference on Machine Learning and Applications, ICMLA '09, pp. 710–714. IEEE Computer Society, Washington, DC (2009)
35. Russell, J.: Affective space is bipolar. J. Pers. Soc. Psychol. **37**, 345–356 (1979)
36. Russell, J.: Core affect and the psychological construction of emotion. Psychol. Rev. **110**, 145–172 (2003)
37. Scherer, K.: Psychological models of emotion. The Neuropsychology of Emotion Pages, pp. 137–162 (2000)
38. Slaughter, L.: Semantic relationships in health consumer questions and physicians answers: a basis for representing medical knowledge and for concept exploration interfaces. Doctoral dissertation, University of Maryland at College Park (2002)
39. Smith, B., Fellbaum, C.: Medical wordnet: a new methodology for the construction and validation of information resources for consumer health. In: Proceedings of the 20th International Conference on Computational Linguistics, COLING '04. Association for Computational Linguistics, Stroudsburg (2004). https://doi.org/10.3115/1220355.1220409
40. Smith, C., Stavri, P., Chapman, W.: In their own words? A terminological analysis of e-mail to a cancer information service. In: Proceedings of AMIA Symposium, p. 697 (2002)
41. Turney, P.D.: Thumbs up or thumbs down? Semantic orientation applied to unsupervised classification of reviews. CoRR cs.LG/0212032 (2002)
42. UzZaman, N., Allen, J.F.: Event and temporal expression extraction from raw text: first step towards a temporally aware system. Int. J. Semantic Computing **4**(4), 487–508 (2010). http://doi.org/10.1142/S1793351X10001097
43. Whissell, C.: The dictionary of affect in language. Emot. Theory Res. Exp. **4**, 113–131 (1989)
44. Wilson, T., Wiebe, J., Hoffman, P.: Recognizing contextual polarity in phrase level sentiment analysis. ACL **7**(5), 12–21 (2005)
45. Wilson, T., Wiebe, J., Hwa, R.: Just how mad are you? Finding strong and weak opinion clauses. In: AAAI, San Jose, pp. 761–769 (2004)

Chapter 3
SenticNet

Abstract SenticNet is the knowledge base the sentic computing framework leverages on for concept-level sentiment analysis. This chapter illustrates how such a resource is built. In particular, the chapter thoroughly explains the processes of knowledge acquisition, representation, and reasoning, which contribute to the generation of the semantics and sentics that form SenticNet. This chapter describes the knowledge bases and knowledge sources SenticNet is built upon. Then it describes how the knowledge collected is represented in graph, matrix and vector space. Then it dives into the techniques adopted for generating semantics and sentics, finally discussing how the proposed framework outperforms the state-of-the-art methods.

Keywords Knowledge representation and reasoning • Semantic network • Vector space model • Spreading activation • Emotion categorization • Sentic computing

SenticNet [22] is a publicly available semantic resource for concept-level sentiment analysis that exploits an ensemble of graph-mining and dimensionality-reduction techniques to bridge the conceptual and affective gap between word-level natural language data and the concept-level opinions and sentiments conveyed by them [29]. SenticNet is a knowledge base that can be employed for the development of applications in fields such as big social data analysis, human-computer interaction, and e-health. It is available either as a standalone XML repository[1] or as an API.[2]

SenticNet provides the semantics and sentics associated with 50,000 common-sense concepts, instantiated by either single words or multi-word expressions. A full list of such concepts is available at http://sentic.net/api/en/concept. Other API methods include http://sentic.net/api/en/concept/CONCEPT_NAME, to retrieve all the available information associated with a specific concept, and more fine-grained methods to get semantics, sentics, and polarity, respectively:

---

[1]http://sentic.net/senticnet-4.0.zip

[2]http://sentic.net/api

© Springer International Publishing AG 2017

R. Satapathy et al., *Sentiment Analysis in the Bio-Medical Domain*,
Socio-Affective Computing 7, https://doi.org/10.1007/978-3-319-68468-0_3

1. http://sentic.net/api/en/concept/CONCEPT_NAME/semantics
2. http://sentic.net/api/en/concept/CONCEPT_NAME/sentics
3. http://sentic.net/api/en/concept/CONCEPT_NAME/polarity
4. http://sentic.net/api/en/concept/CONCEPT_NAME/moodtags

In particular, the first command returns five SenticNet entries that are semantically related to the input concept, the second provides four affective values in
terms of the dimensions of the Hourglass of Emotions (Sect. 3.3.2), and the third
returns a float number between −1 and 1, which is calculated in terms of the sentics
and specifies if (and to which extent) the input concept is positive or negative. The
fourth provides the moodtags by using Hourglass model. For example, the full set
of conceptual features associated with the multi-word expression `cry_baby` can
be retrieved with the following API call (Fig. 3.1): http://sentic.net/api/en/concept/
cry_baby

In case only the semantics associated with `cry_baby` are needed, e.g., for
gisting or auto-categorization tasks, these can be obtained by simply appending
the command *semantics* to the above (Fig. 3.2). Similarly, the sentics associated
with `cry_baby`, useful for tasks such as affective HCI or theory of mind, can

```
▼<rdf:RDF xmlns:rdf="http://w3.org/1999/02/22-rdf-syntax-ns#">
 ▼<rdf:Description rdf:about="http://sentic.net/api/en/concept/cry_baby">
   <rdf:type rdf:resource="http://sentic.net/api/en/concept/"/>
   <text xmlns="http://sentic.net">cry baby</text>
  ▼<semantics xmlns="http://sentic.net">
    <concept xmlns="http://sentic.net" rdf:resource="http://sentic.net/api/en/concept/bad_music"/>
    <concept xmlns="http://sentic.net" rdf:resource="http://sentic.net/api/en/concept/noise"/>
    <concept xmlns="http://sentic.net" rdf:resource="http://sentic.net/api/en/concept/stress"/>
    <concept xmlns="http://sentic.net" rdf:resource="http://sentic.net/api/en/concept/a_lot_of_work"/>
    <concept xmlns="http://sentic.net" rdf:resource="http://sentic.net/api/en/concept/stressful_situation"/>
   </semantics>
  ▼<sentics xmlns="http://sentic.net">
    <pleasantness xmlns="http://sentic.net" rdf:datatype="http://w3.org/2001/XMLSchema#float">0.062</pleasantness>
    <attention xmlns="http://sentic.net" rdf:datatype="http://w3.org/2001/XMLSchema#float">-0.03</attention>
    <sensitivity xmlns="http://sentic.net" rdf:datatype="http://w3.org/2001/XMLSchema#float">0.116</sensitivity>
    <aptitude xmlns="http://sentic.net" rdf:datatype="http://w3.org/2001/XMLSchema#float">-0.09</aptitude>
   </sentics>
  ▼<moodtags xmlns="http://sentic.net">
    <concept xmlns="http://sentic.net" rdf:resource="http://sentic.net/api/en/concept/anger"/>
    <concept xmlns="http://sentic.net" rdf:resource="http://sentic.net/api/en/concept/disgust"/>
   </moodtags>
  ▼<polarity xmlns="http://sentic.net">
    <value xmlns="http://sentic.net">negative</value>
    <intensity xmlns="http://sentic.net" rdf:datatype="http://w3.org/2001/XMLSchema#float">-0.03</intensity>
   </polarity>
  </rdf:Description>
 </rdf:RDF>
```

Fig. 3.1 Sentic API concept call sample (Source: http://sentic.net/api)

```
▼<rdf:RDF xmlns:rdf="http://w3.org/1999/02/22-rdf-syntax-ns#">
 ▼<rdf:Description rdf:about="http://sentic.net/api/en/concept/cry_baby/semantics">
   <rdf:type rdf:resource="http://sentic.net/api/en/concept/semantics"/>
  ▼<semantics xmlns="http://sentic.net">
    <concept xmlns="http://sentic.net" rdf:resource="http://sentic.net/api/en/concept/bad_music"/>
    <concept xmlns="http://sentic.net" rdf:resource="http://sentic.net/api/en/concept/noise"/>
    <concept xmlns="http://sentic.net" rdf:resource="http://sentic.net/api/en/concept/stress"/>
    <concept xmlns="http://sentic.net" rdf:resource="http://sentic.net/api/en/concept/a_lot_of_work"/>
    <concept xmlns="http://sentic.net" rdf:resource="http://sentic.net/api/en/concept/stressful_situation"/>
   </semantics>
  </rdf:Description>
 </rdf:RDF>
```

Fig. 3.2 Sentic API concept semantics call (Source: hhttp://sentic.net/api/en/concept/cry_baby/
semantics)

```
▼<rdf:RDF xmlns:rdf="http://w3.org/1999/02/22-rdf-syntax-ns#">
  ▼<rdf:Description rdf:about="http://sentic.net/api/en/concept/cry_baby/sentics">
    <rdf:type rdf:resource="http://sentic.net/api/concept/sentics"/>
  ▼<sentics xmlns="http://sentic.net">
    <pleasantness xmlns="http://sentic.net" rdf:datatype="http://www.w3.org/2001/XMLSchema#float">0.062</pleasantness>
    <attention xmlns="http://sentic.net" rdf:datatype="http://www.w3.org/2001/XMLSchema#float">-0.03</attention>
    <sensitivity xmlns="http://sentic.net" rdf:datatype="http://www.w3.org/2001/XMLSchema#float">0.116</sensitivity>
    <aptitude xmlns="http://sentic.net" rdf:datatype="http://www.w3.org/2001/XMLSchema#float">-0.09</aptitude>
    </sentics>
  </rdf:Description>
</rdf:RDF>
```

Fig. 3.3 Sentic API concept sentics call (Source: http://sentic.net/api/en/concept/cry_baby/sentics)

```
▼<rdf:RDF xmlns:rdf="http://w3.org/1999/02/22-rdf-syntax-ns#">
  ▼<rdf:Description rdf:about="http://sentic.net/api/en/concept/cry_baby/moodtag">
    <rdf:type rdf:resource="http://sentic.net/api/concept/moodtag"/>
  ▼<moodtags xmlns="http://sentic.net">
    <concept xmlns="http://sentic.net" rdf:resource="http://sentic.net/api/en/concept/anger"/>
    <concept xmlns="http://sentic.net" rdf:resource="http://sentic.net/api/en/concept/disgust"/>
    </moodtags>
  </rdf:Description>
</rdf:RDF>
```

Fig. 3.4 Sentic API concept moodtags call (Source: http://sentic.net/api/en/concept/cry_baby/moodtags)

```
▼<rdf:RDF xmlns:rdf="http://w3.org/1999/02/22-rdf-syntax-ns#">
  ▼<rdf:Description rdf:about="http://sentic.net/api/en/concept/cry_baby/polarity">
    <rdf:type rdf:resource="http://sentic.net/api/concept/polarity"/>
  ▼<polarity xmlns="http://sentic.net">
    <value xmlns="http://sentic.net">negative</value>
    <intensity xmlns="http://sentic.net" rdf:datatype="http://www.w3.org/2001/XMLSchema#float">-0.03</intensity>
    </polarity>
  </rdf:Description>
</rdf:RDF>
```

Fig. 3.5 Sentic API concept polarity call (Source: http://sentic.net/api/en/concept/cry_baby/polarity)

be retrieved by adding the command *sentics* (Fig. 3.3). Sentics can be converted to emotion labels, e.g., 'anger' and 'disgust' in this case, by using the Hourglass model (Fig. 3.4).

Finally, the polarity associated with `cry_baby`, which can be exploited for more standard sentiment analysis tasks, can be obtained through the command *polarity* (Fig. 3.5).

Unlike many other sentiment analysis resources, SenticNet is not built by manually labeling pieces of knowledge coming from general NLP resources such as WordNet or DBPedia. Instead, it is automatically constructed by applying graph-mining and multi-dimensional scaling techniques on the affective commonsense knowledge collected from three different sources (Sect. 3.1). This knowledge is represented redundantly at three levels: semantic network, matrix, and vector space (Sect. 3.2). Subsequently, semantics and sentics are calculated though the ensemble application of spreading activation, neural networks and an emotion categorization model (Sect. 3.3). The SenticNet construction framework (Fig. 3.6) merges all these techniques and models together in order to generate a knowledge base of 30,000 concepts and a set of semantics, sentics, and polarity for each of them.

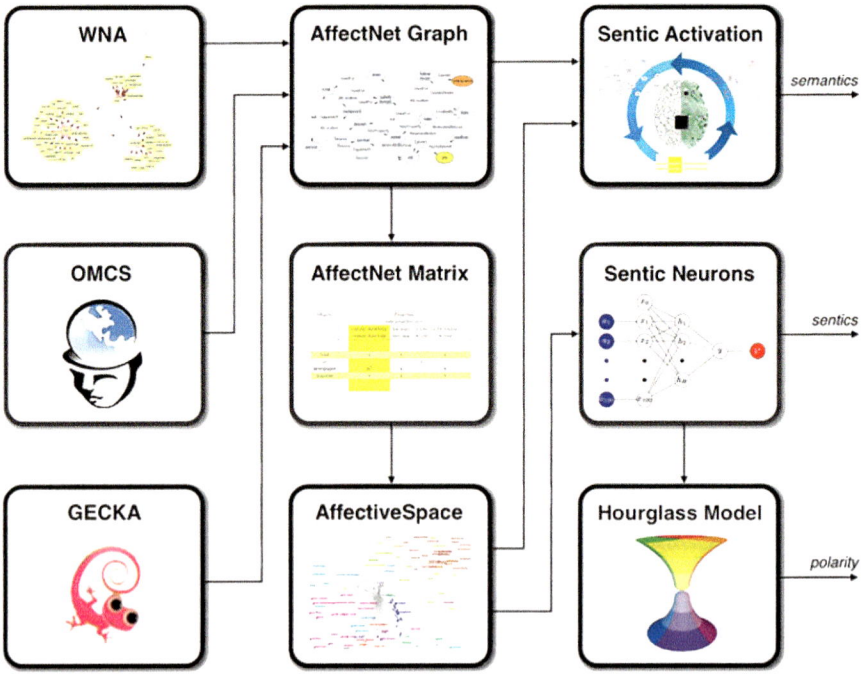

Fig. 3.6 SenticNet construction framework: by leveraging on an ensemble of graph mining and multi-dimensional scaling techniques, this framework generates the semantics and sentics that form the SenticNet knowledge base (Source: Sentic Computing [22])

3.1   Knowledge Acquisition

This section describes the knowledge bases and knowledge sources SenticNet is built upon. SenticNet mainly leverages on the general commonsense knowledge extracted from the Open Mind Common Sense initiative (Sect. 3.1.1), the affective knowledge coming from WordNet-Affect (Sect. 3.1.2) and the practical commonsense knowledge crowdsourced from GECKA (Sect. 3.1.3).

3.1.1   Open Mind Common Sense

Open Mind Common Sense (OMCS) is an AI project based at the MIT Media Lab whose goal is to build and utilize a large commonsense knowledge base from the contributions of many thousands of people across the Web.

Since its founding in 1999, it has accumulated more than a million English facts from over 15,000 contributors in addition to knowledge bases in other languages. The project was the brainchild of Marvin Minsky, Push Singh, and Catherine

Havasi. Development work began in September 1999, and the project was opened to the Internet a year later. Havasi described it in her dissertation as "an attempt to ...harness some of the distributed human computing power of the Internet, an idea which was then only in its early stages" [46]. The original OMCS was influenced by the website Everything2, a collaborative Web-based community consisting of a database of interlinked user-submitted written material, and presented a minimalist interface that was inspired by Google.

There are many different types of knowledge in OMCS. Some statements convey relationships between objects or events, expressed as simple phrases of natural language: some examples include "A coat is used for keeping warm", "The sun is very hot", and "The last thing you do when you cook dinner is wash your dishes". The database also contains information on the emotional content of situations, in such statements as "Spending time with friends causes happiness" and "Getting into a car wreck makes one angry". OMCS contains information on people's desires and goals, both large and small, such as "People want to be respected" and "People want good coffee" [99]. Originally, these statements could be entered into the Web site as unconstrained sentences of text, which had to be parsed later. The current version of the Web site collects knowledge only using more structured fill-in-the-blank templates. OMCS also makes use of data collected by the Game With a Purpose "Verbosity" [6].

OMCS differs from Cyc because it has focused on representing the commonsense knowledge it collected as English sentences, rather than using a formal logical structure. Due to its emphasis on informal conceptual-connectedness over formal linguistic-rigor, OMCS knowledge is structured more like WordNet than Cyc. In its native form, the OMCS database is simply a collection of these short sentences that convey some common knowledge. In order to use this knowledge computationally, it has to be transformed into a more structured representation.

3.1.2 WordNet-Affect

WordNet-Affect (WNA) [100] is an extension of WordNet Domains, including a subset of synsets suitable to represent affective concepts correlated with affective words. Similarly to the method used for domain labels, a number of WordNet synsets is assigned to one or more affective labels (a-labels). In particular, the affective concepts representing emotional state are individuated by synsets marked with the a-label emotion. There are also other a-labels for those concepts representing moods, situations eliciting emotions, or emotional responses. The resource was extended with a set of additional a-labels (called emotional categories), hierarchically organized, in order to specialize synsets with a-label emotion. The hierarchical structure of new a-labels was modeled on the WordNet hyperonym relation.

Table 3.1 A-labels and corresponding example synsets (Source: http://wndomains.fbk.eu/wnaffect.html)

A-labels	Examples
Emotion	Noun anger#1, verb fear#1
Mood	Noun animosisy#1, adjective amiable#1
Trait	Noun aggressiveness#1, adjective competitive#1
Cognitive state	Noun confusion#2, adjective dazed#2
Physical state	Noun illness#1, adjective all in#1
Hedonic signal	Noun hurt#3, noun suffering#4
Emotion-eliciting situation	Noun awkwardness#3, adjective out of danger#1
Emotional response	Noun cold sweat#1, verb tremble#2
Behavior	Noun offense#1, adjective inhibited#1
Attitude	Noun intolerance#1, noun defensive#1
Sensation	Noun coldness#1, verb feel#3

In a second stage, some modifications were introduced, in order to distinguish synsets according to emotional valence. Four additional a-labels were defined: positive, negative, ambiguous, and neutral (Table 3.1). The first one corresponds to positive emotions, defined as emotional states characterized by the presence of positive edonic signals (or pleasure). It includes synsets such as joy#1 or enthusiasm#1. Similarly the negative a-label identifies negative emotions characterized by negative edonic signals (or pain), for example anger#1 or sadness#1. Synsets representing affective states whose valence depends on semantic context (e.g., surprise#1) were marked with the tag ambiguous. Finally, synsets referring to mental states that are generally considered affective but are not characterized by valence, were marked with the tag neutral.

Another important property for affective lexicon concerning mainly adjectival interpretation is the stative/causative dimension. An emotional adjective is said causative if it refers to some emotion that is caused by the entity represented by the modified noun (e.g., amusing movie). In a similar way, an emotional adjective is said stative if it refers to the emotion owned or felt by the subject denoted by the modified noun (e.g., cheerful/happy boy).

All words can potentially convey affective meaning. Each of them, even those more apparently neutral, can evoke pleasant or painful experiences. While some words have emotional meaning with respect to the individual story, for many others the affective power is part of the collective imagination (e.g., words mum, ghost, war etc.). Therefore, it is interesting to individuate a way to measure the affective meaning of a generic term. To this aim, the use of words in textual productions was studied, and in particular their co-occurrences with the words in which the affective meaning is explicit. It is necessary to distinguish between words directly referring to emotional states (e.g., fear, cheerful) and those having only an indirect reference that depends on the context (e.g., words that indicate possible emotional causes as monster or emotional responses as cry). The former are termed 'direct affective words' and the latter 'indirect affective words'.

Direct affective words were first integrated in WNA; then, a selection function (named Affective-Weight) based on a semantic similarity mechanism automatically acquired in an unsupervised way from a large corpus of texts (100 millions of words) was applied in order to individuate the indirect affective lexicon. Applied to a concept (e.g., a WordNet synset) and an emotional category, this function returns a value representing the semantic affinity with that emotion. In this way it is possible to assign a value to the concept with respect to each emotional category, and eventually select the emotion with the highest value. Applied to a set of concepts that are semantically similar, this function selects subsets characterized by some given affective constraints (e.g., referring to a particular emotional category or valence).

Authors were able to focus selectively on positive, negative, ambiguous or neutral types of emotions. For example, given difficulty as input term, the system suggests as related emotions (a-labels): identification, negative-concern, ambiguous-expectation, apathy. Moreover, given an input word (e.g., university) and the indication of an emotional valence (e.g., positive), the system suggests a set of related words through some positive emotional category (e.g., professor, scholarship, achievement) found through the emotions enthusiasm, sympathy, devotion, encouragement. These fine-grained kinds of affective lexicon selection can open up new possibilities in many applications that exploit verbal communication of emotions.

3.1.3   GECKA

Games with a purpose (GWAPs) are a simple yet powerful means to collect useful information from players in a way that is entertaining for them. Over the past few years, GWAPs have sought to exploit the brainpower made available by multitudes of casual gamers to perform tasks that, despite being relatively easy for humans to complete, are rather unfeasible for machines. The key idea is to integrate tasks such as image tagging, video annotation, and text classification into games, [3] producing win-win situations where people have fun while actually doing something useful. These games focus on exploiting player input to (syntax, not: both create) create both meaningful data and provide more enjoyable game experiences [101]. The problem with current GWAPs is that information gathered from them is often unrecyclable; acquired data is often applicable only to the specific stimuli encountered during gameplay. Moreover, such games often have a fairly low 'sticky factor', and are often unable to engage gamers for more than a few minutes.

GECKA (game engine for commonsense knowledge acquisition) [30] implements a new GWAP concept that aims to overcome the main drawbacks of traditional data-collecting games by empowering users to create their own GWAPs and by mining knowledge that is highly reusable and multi-purpose. In particular, GECKA allows users to design compelling serious games for their peers to play and, while doing so, gather commonsense knowledge useful for intelligent applications in any field requiring in-depth knowledge of the real world, including reasoning, perception and social systems simulation.

Besides allowing for the acquisition of knowledge from game designers, GECKA enables players of the finished games to be educated in useful ways, all while being entertained. The knowledge gained from GECKA is later encoded in AffecNet in the form <concept-relationship-concept>. The use of this natural language based (rather than logic-based) framework allows GECKA players to conceptualize the world in their own terms, at an ideal level of semantic abstraction. Players can work with knowledge exactly as they envision it, and researchers can access data on the same level as players' thoughts, greatly enhancing the usefulness of the captured data.

3.1.3.1   GWAP

GWAPs are an example of an emerging class of games that can be considered 'human algorithms', since humans act as processing nodes for problems that computers cannot yet solve. By providing an incentive for players, GWAPs gain a large quantity of computing power that can be harnessed for multiple applications, e.g., content tagging, ontology building, and knowledge acquisition by the general public.

GWAPs are possibly most famous for image annotation. In the 'ESP' game [4], for example, players guess content objects or properties of random images by typing what they see when it appears on the screen. Other image annotation games include: Matchin [45], which focuses on perceived image quality by asking players to pairwise choose the picture they like better, and Phetch [5], a game that collects explanatory descriptions of images in order to improve Web accessibility for the visually impaired. Peekaboom [7] focuses on locating objects within images by letting a player select and reveal specific parts of an image and then challenging the other to guess the correct object name, while Squigl challenges players to spot objects in images previously annotated within the ESP Game. 'Picture This' requires players to choose from a set of images the one that best suits the given query. Image annotation games also include those intended to help streamline the robustness of CAPTCHAs, such as Magic Bullet [107], a team game in which players need to agree on the meaning of CAPTCHAs, and TagCaptcha [79], where players are asked to quickly describe CAPTCHA images with single words.

Besides images, GWAPs have been used for video annotation. For example, OntoTube [94], Yahoo's Videotaggame [109], and Waisd [2], are all games in which two players have to quickly agree on a set of tags for the same streaming YouTube video. GWAPs have also been exploited to automatically tag music tracks with semantic labels. HerdIt [11], for example, asks players to accomplish various tasks and answer quizzes related to the song they are listening to. In Tagatune [61], two players listen to an audio file and describe to the other what they are hearing. Players must then decide whether or not the game has played the same soundtrack to both participants. Sophisticated GWAPs have also attempted to perform complex tasks such as Web-page annotation and ontology building. Page Hunt [71], for example, is a GWAP that shows players Web pages and asks the user to guess what queries would generate those pages within the top five hits.

Results are used to improve the Microsoft Bing search engine. The game then shows players the top five page hits for the entered keywords and rewards are granted depending on how highly-ranked the assigned Web pages are within the result set. Another example, OntoPronto [94], is a quiz game for vocabulary building that attempts to build a large domain ontology from Wikipedia articles. Players receive random articles, which they map to the most specific appropriate class of the Proton ontology (using the *subClassOf* relationship).

Another interesting game for generating domain ontologies from open data is Guess What?! [74]. Given a seed concept, a player has to find the matching URI in DBpedia, Freebase and OpenCyc. The resulting labels/URIs are analyzed by simple computer-game-design tools in order to identify expressions that can be translated into logical operators, breaking down complex descriptions into small fragments. The game starts with the most general fragment and, at each round, a more specific fragment is connected to it through a logical operator, with players having to guess the concept described. Other GWAPs aim to align ontologies. Wordhunger, for example, is a Web-based application mapping WordNet synsets to Freebase. Each game round consists of a WordNet term and up to three suggested possible Freebase articles, among which players have to select the most fitting.

SpotTheLink is a two player game focusing on the alignment of random concepts from the DBpedia Ontology to the Proton upper ontology. Each player has to select Proton concepts that are either the same as, or, more specific than a randomly selected DBpedia concept. Data generated by SpotTheLink generates a SKOS mapping between the concepts of the two input ontologies. Finally, Wikiracing, Wiki Game, Wikispeedia and WikipediaMaze are games which aim to improve Wikipedia by engaging gamers in finding connections between articles by clicking links within article texts. WikipediaGame and Wikispedia focus on completing the race faster and with fewer clicks than other players. On the other hand, WikipediaMaze allows players to create races for each other and are incentivized to create and play races through the possibility of earning badges.

One of the most interesting tasks GWAPs can be used for is commonsense knowledge acquisition from members of the general public. One example, Verbosity [6], is a real time quiz game for collecting commonsense facts. In the game, two players take different roles at different times: one functions as a narrator, who has to describe a word using templates, while the other has to guess the word in the shortest time possible. FACTory Game [65] is a GWAP developed by Cycorp which randomly chooses facts from Cyc and presents them to players in order for them to guess whether a statement is true, false, or does not make sense. A variant of the FACTory game is the Concept Game on Facebook [49], which collects commonsense knowledge by proposing random assertions to users (along the lines of a slot machine) and gets them to decide whether the given assertion is meaningful or not. Virtual Pet [59] aims to construct a semantic network that encodes commonsense knowledge, and is built upon PPT, a popular Chinese bulletin board system accessible through a terminal interface. In this game each player owns a pet, which they take care of by asking and answering questions.

The pet acts as a stand-in for other players who then receive these questions and answers, and have to respond to or validate them. Similar to Virtual Pet, the Rapport Game [59] draws on player efforts in constructing a semantic network that encodes commonsense knowledge. The Rapport Game, however, is built on top of Facebook and uses direct interaction between players. Finally, the Hourglass Game [31] is a timed game that associates natural language concepts with affective labels on a hourglass-shaped emotion categorization model. Players not only earn points in accordance with the accuracy of their associations, but also for their speed in creating affective matches. The game is able to collect new pieces of affective commonsense knowledge by randomly proposing multi-word expressions for which no affective information is known. The aggregation of this information generates a list of affective commonsense concepts, each weighted by a confidence score proportional to an inter-annotator agreement, which is therefore highly useful for opinion mining and sentiment analysis.

3.1.3.2   GECKA Key Functionalities

An important difference between traditional artificial intelligence (AI) systems and human intelligence is the human ability to harness commonsense knowledge gleaned from a lifetime of learning and experience to make informed decisions. This allows humans to adapt easily to novel situations where AI fails catastrophically due to a lack of situation-specific rules and generalization capabilities. Commonsense knowledge also provides background information enabling humans to successfully operate in social situations where such knowledge is typically assumed.

Distributed online knowledge acquisition projects have become quite popular in the past years. Examples include: Freebase,[3] NELL,[4] and ProBase.[5] Other examples include the different projects associated with the Open Mind Initiative, e.g., OMCS, Open Mind Indoor Common Sense [44], which aims to develop intelligent mobile robots for use in home and office environments, and Open Mind Common Sentics [31], a set of GWAPs for the acquisition of affective commonsense knowledge used to enrich SenticNet.

Whereas previous approaches have relied on paid experts or unpaid volunteers, GECKA puts a much stronger emphasis on creating a system that is appealing to a large audience, regardless of whether or not they are interested in contributing to AI. The fundamental aim of GECKA is to transform the activity of entering knowledge into an enjoyable, interactive process as much as possible. Most GWAPs today may be fun to play for a relatively short period of time, but players are not often keen on

---

[3] http://freebase.com

[4] http://rtw.ml.cmu.edu/rtw

[5] http://research.microsoft.com/probase

returning. It goes to say that GWAPs generally evidence a fairly low 'sticky factor', defined as the amount of daily active users (DAUs) of an application divided by the number of monthly active users (MAUs).

While MAU on its own is the most-quoted measure of a game's size, it is only effective in describing size or reach, and not engagement. Similarly, DAU can be a very valuable metric, given that it indicates how much activity a game sees on a daily basis. However, it falls into the same trap as MAU in that it does not discriminate between player-base retention and acquisition. The single-most important metric for engagement is stickiness, i.e., DAU/MAU, which enables more accurate calculation of repeat visits and average knowledge acquired per user (AKAPU).

The key to enhancing a game's sticky factor, besides great gameplay, is the ability of an application to prompt users to reach out to their friends, e.g., via stories and pictures about their gameplay. To this end, GECKA allows users to design compelling serious games that can be made available on the App Store for their peers to play (Fig. 3.7). As opposed to traditional GWAPs, GECKA does not limit users to specific, often boring, tasks, but rather gives them the freedom to choose both the kind and the granularity of knowledge to be encoded, through a user-friendly and intuitive interface. This not only improves gameplay and game-stickiness, but also allows commonsense knowledge to be collected in ways that are not predictable a priori.

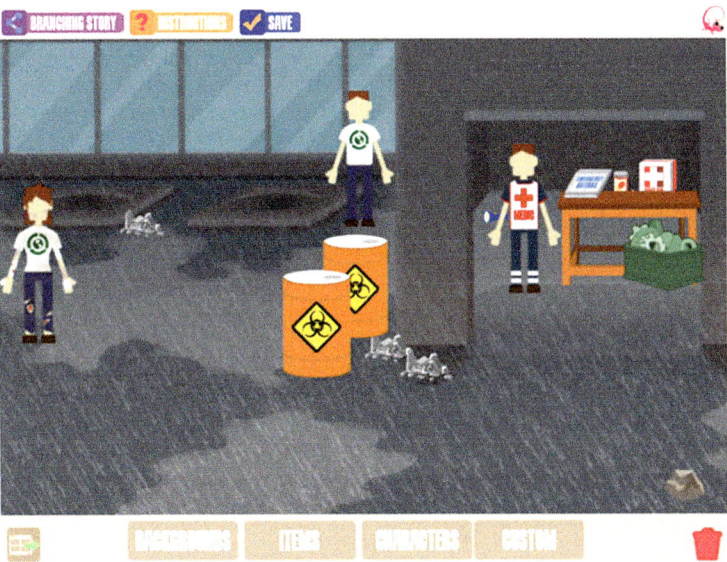

Fig. 3.7 Outdoor scenario. Game designers can drag&drop objects and characters from the library and specify how these interact with each other (Source: [30])

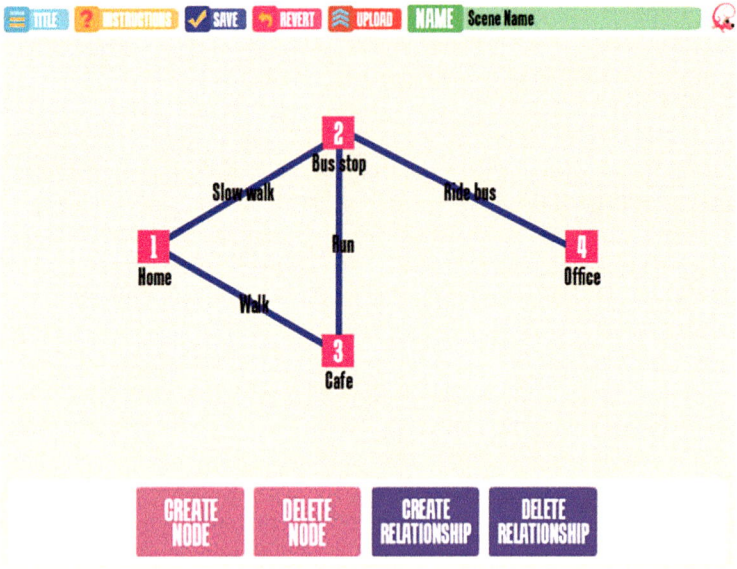

Fig. 3.8 Branching story screen. Game designers can name and connect different scenes according to their semantics and role in the story of the game (Source: [30])

Not just a system for the creation of microgames, GECKA is a serious game engine that aims to give designers the means to create long adventure games to be played by others. To this end, GECKA offers functionalities typical of role-play games (RPGs), e.g., a question/answer dialogue box enabling communication and the exchange of objects (optionally tied to correct answers) between players and virtual world inhabitants, a library for enriching scenes with useful and yet visually-appealing objects, backgrounds, characters, and a branching storyline for defining how different game scenes are interconnected.

In the branching story screen, game designers place scene nodes and connect them by defining semantic conditions that specify how the player will move from a scene to another (Fig. 3.8). Making a scene transition may require fulfillment of a complex goal, acquisition of an object, or some other relevant condition. These conditions provide invaluable information about the prerequisites of certain actions and the objects that participate in action and goal flows. Goals are created by the combination of smaller semantic primitives ('can', 'cannot', actions, places, and so on), enabling users to specify highly nuanced goals.

Designers can associate goal sequences with each story node through the combination of a set of primitives, actions, objects, and emotions (selected from the library) that describe the end state of the world once the goal sequence is complete. The branching story screen aims to acquire transitional commonsense knowledge, e.g., "if I was at the bus stop before and I am now at the office, I am likely to have taken the bus" and situational commonsense knowledge, e.g., "if you are waiting at the bus stop, your goal is probably to reach a different place".

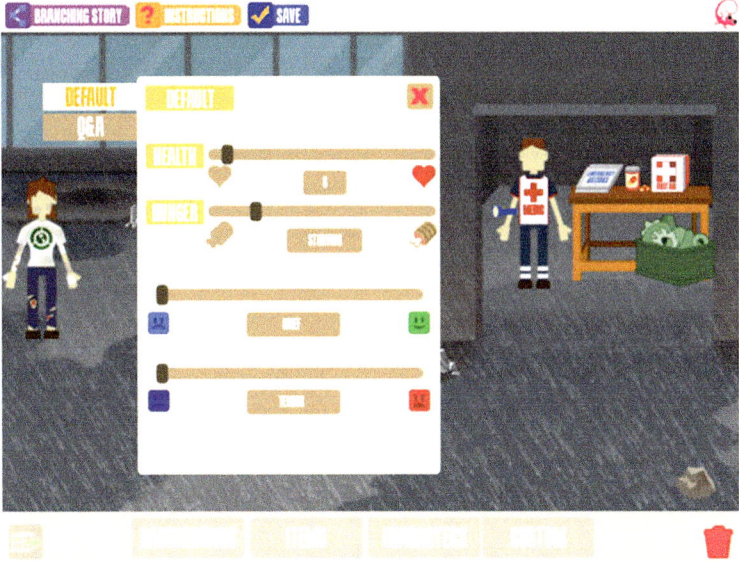

Fig. 3.9 Status of a new character in the scene who is ill and extremely hungry, plus has very low levels of pleasantness (grief) and sensitivity (terror) (Source: [30])

In case an action or an object are not available in the library, GECKA allows game designers to define their own custom items by building shapes from a set of predefined geometric forms or applying transforms to existing items. This enables the creation of new objects for which there is no available icon by combining available graphics and predefined shapes, and the use of transformations to create various object states, such as a 'broken jar'. The ability of users to create their own custom items and actions is key to maintaining an undisrupted game flow. Although the aesthetics of a custom object may not be the same as predefined icons, custom objects allow game designers to express their creativity without limiting themselves to the set of available graphics and, hence, allow researchers to discover new commonsense concepts and the semantic features associated with them (Fig. 3.9).

Whenever game designers create a new object or action, they must specify its name and its semantics through prerequisite-outcome-goal (POG) triples, Prerequisites indicate what must be present or have been done before using the object or action. Outcomes include objects or states of the world (including emotional states, e.g., "if I give money to someone, their happiness is likely to rise"). Goals in turn specify the specific scene goals that are facilitated by that particular POG triple. Game designers drag and drop objects and characters from action/object libraries into scenes. For each object, in particular, they can specify a POG triple that describes how such an object is affected by the actions performed over it (Fig. 3.10). POG triples give us pieces of commonsense information like "if I use a can opener on a can, I obtain the content of the can" or "the result of squeezing an orange, is orange juice".

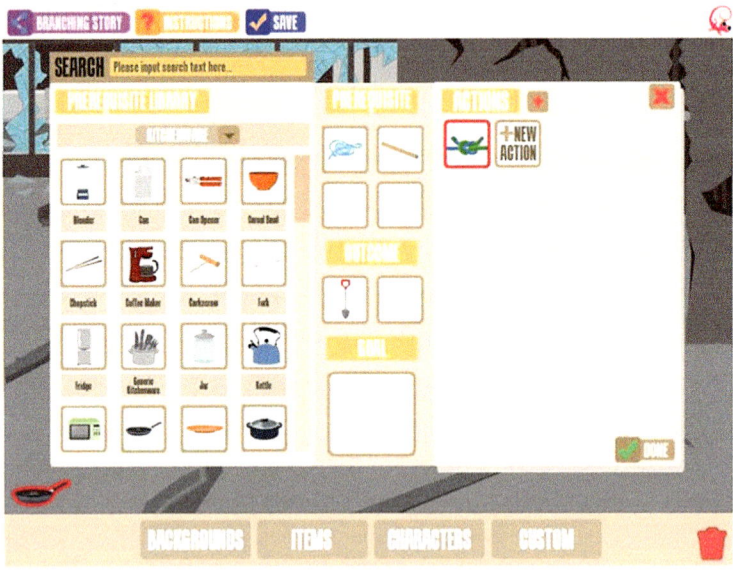

Fig. 3.10 Specification of a POG triple. By applying the action 'tie' over a 'pan', in combination with 'stick' and 'lace', a shovel can be obtained (Source: [30])

Towards the goal of improving gameplay, and because GECKA mainly aims to collect in typical commonsense knowledge, POG triples associated with a specific object type are shared among all the instances of such an object ('inheritance'). Whenever a game designer associates a POG to an object in the scene, that POG instantly becomes shared among all the other objects of the same type, no matter if these are located in different scenes. New instances inherit this POG as well.

Game designers, however, can create exceptions of any object type through the creation of new custom objects. A 'moldy bread' custom object, for example, normally inherits all the POGs of 'bread' but these can be changed, modified, or removed at the time of object instantiation without affecting other 'bread' type objects. The POG specification is among the most effective means to collect commonsense knowledge, given that it is performed quite often by the game designer during the creation of scenes (Fig. 3.11).

From a simple POG definition we may obtain a large amount of knowledge, including interaction semantics between different objects, prerequisites of actions, and the goals commonly associated with such actions (Table 3.2). These pieces of commonsense knowledge, are very clearly-structured, and thus easy to assimilate into the knowledge base, due to the fixed framework for defining interaction semantics. POG specifications not only allow game designers to define interaction semantics between objects but also to specify how the original player, action/object recipients, and non-recipients react to various actions by setting parameters involving character health, hunger, pleasantness, and sensitivity (Fig. 3.9). While the first

```
<scenes>
    <sceneData>
        <sceneType>
            <string>kitchen</string>
        </sceneType>
        <items>
            <itemData>
                <itemType>
                    <string>bread slices</string>
                </itemType>
                <position>
                    <x>8.04757</x>
                    <y>2.32971239</y>
                </position>
                <actions>
                    <actionData>
                        <actionType>
                            <string>stack</string>
                        </actionType>
                        <POG_Data>
                            <prerequisites>
                                <string>ham</string>
                                <string>mayonnaise</string>
                            </prerequisites>
                            <outcomes>
                                <string>sandwich</string>
                            </outcomes>
                            <goal>
                                <string>satisfy hunger</string>
                            </goal>
                        </POG_Data>
                        <player>
                            <affect>
                                <health>80</health>
                                <hunger>50</hunger>
                                <pleasantness>5</pleasantness>
                                <sensitivity>3</sensitivity>
                            </affect>
                        </player>
                        <recipientCharacter>
                            <type>hungry man</type>
                            <affect>
                                <health>80</health>
                                <hunger>50</hunger>
                                <pleasantness>5</pleasantness>
                                <sensitivity>3</sensitivity>
                            </affect>
                        </recipientCharacter>
                        <nonRecipientCharacter>
```

Fig. 3.11 A sample XML output deriving from the creation of a scene in GECKA. Actions are collected and encoded according to their semantics (Source: [30])

two parameters allow more physiological commonsense knowledge to be collected, pleasantness and sensitivity directly map affective commonsense knowledge onto the Hourglass model. This is, in turn, used to enhance reasoning within SenticNet, especially for tasks such as emotion recognition, goal inference, and sentiment analysis.

Table 3.2 List of most common POG triples collected during a pilot testing (Source: [30])

Item	Action	Prerequisite	Outcome	Goal
Orange	Squeeze	–	Orange juice	Quench thirst
Bread	Cut	Knife	Bread slices	–
Bread slices	Stack	Ham, mayonnaise	Sandwich	Satisfy hunger
Coffee beans	Hit	Pestle	Coffee powder	–
Coffee maker	Fill	Coffee powder, water	Coffee	–
Bottle	Fill	Water	Bottled water	Quench thirst
Chair	Hit	Hammer	Wood pieces	–
Can	Open	Can opener	Food	Satisfy hunger
Towel	Cut	Scissors	Bandage	–
Sack	Fill	Sand	Sandbag	Flood control

3.2   Knowledge Representation

This section describes how the knowledge collected from OMCS, WNA, and
GECKA is represented redundantly at three levels: semantic network, matrix, and
vector space. In particular, the collected or crowdsourced pieces of knowledge
are firstly integrated in a semantic network as triples of the format <concept-
relationship-concept> (Sect. 3.2.1). Secondly, the graph is represented as a matrix
having concepts as rows and the combination <relationship-concept> as columns
(Sect. 3.2.1). Finally, multi-dimensionality reduction is applied to such a matrix
in order to create a vector space representation of commonsense knowledge
(Sect. 3.2.3).

3.2.1   AffectNet Graph

AffectNet is an affective commonsense knowledge base mainly built upon ConceptNet [98], the graph representation of the Open Mind corpus, which structurally
similar to WordNet, but whose scope of contents is general world knowledge, in
the same vein as Cyc. Instead of insisting on formalizing commonsense reasoning
using mathematical logic [80], ConceptNet uses a new approach: it represents
data in the form of a semantic network and makes it available to be used in
natural language processing. The prerogative of ConceptNet, in fact, is contextual
commonsense reasoning: while WordNet is optimized for lexical categorization
and word-similarity determination, and Cyc is optimized for formalized logical
reasoning, ConceptNet is optimized for making practical context-based inferences
over real-world texts.

In ConceptNet, WordNet's notion of node in the semantic network is extended
from purely lexical items (words and simple phrases with atomic meaning) to
include higher-order compound concepts, e.g., 'satisfy hunger' and 'follow recipe',

Table 3.3 Comparison between WordNet and ConceptNet. While WordNet synsets contain vocabulary knowledge, ConceptNet assertions convey knowledge about what concepts are used for (Source: [22])

Term	WordNet hypernyms	ConceptNet assertions
Cat	Feline; Felid; Adult male; Man; Gossip; Gossiper; Gossipmonger; Rumormonger; Rumourmonger; Newsmonger; Woman; Adult female; Stimulant; Stimulant drug; Excitant; Tracked vehicle; …	Cats can hunt mice; Cats have whiskers; Cats can eat mice; Cats have fur; cats have claws; Cats can eat meat; cats are cute; …
Dog	Canine; Canid; Disagreeable woman; Chap; Fellow; Feller; Lad; Gent; Fella; Scoundrel; Sausage; Follow, …	Dogs are mammals; A dog can be a pet; A dog can guard a house; You are likely to find a dog in kennel; An activity a dog can do is run; A dog is a loyal friend; A dog has fur; …
Language	Communication; Auditory communication; Word; Higher cognitive process; Faculty; Mental faculty; Module; Text; Textual matter; …	English is a language; French is a language; Language is used for communication; Music is a language; A word is part of language; …
iPhone	N/A	An iPhone is a kind of telephone; An iPhone is a kind of computer; An IPhone can display your position on a map; An IPhone can send and receive emails; An IPhone can display the time; …
Birthday gift	Present	Card is birthday gift; Present is birthday gift; Buying something for a loved one is for a birthday gift; …

to represent knowledge around a greater range of concepts found in everyday life (Table 3.3). Moreover WordNet's repertoire of semantic relations is extended from the triplet of synonym, *IsA* and *PartOf*, to a repertoire of twenty semantic relations including, for example, *EffectOf* (causality), *SubeventOf* (event hierarchy), *CapableOf* (agent's ability), *MotivationOf* (affect), *PropertyOf*, and *LocationOf*. ConceptNet's knowledge is also of a more informal, defeasible, and practically valued nature (Fig. 3.12).

For example, WordNet has formal taxonomic knowledge that 'dog' is a 'canine', which is a 'carnivore', which is a 'placental mammal'; but it cannot make the practically oriented member-to-set association that 'dog' is a 'pet'. ConceptNet also contains a lot of knowledge that is defeasible, i.e., it describes something that is often true but not always, e.g., EffectOf('fall off bicycle', 'get hurt'), which is something we cannot leave aside in commonsense reasoning. Most of the facts interrelating ConceptNet's semantic network are dedicated to making rather generic connections between concepts. This type of knowledge can be brought back to Minsky's K-lines, as it increases the connectivity of the semantic network and makes it more likely that concepts parsed out of a text document can be mapped into ConceptNet.

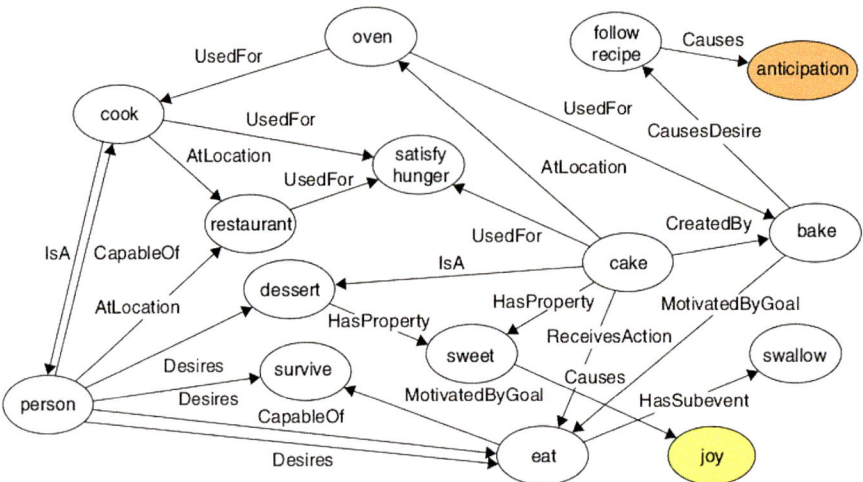

Fig. 3.12 A sketch of the AffectNet graph showing part of the semantic network for the concept cake. The directed graph not only specifies semantic relations between concepts but also connects these to affective nodes (Source: Sentic Computing [22])

ConceptNet is produced by an automatic process, which first applies a set of extraction rules to the semi-structured English sentences of the OMCS corpus, and then applies an additional set of 'relaxation' procedures, i.e., filling in and smoothing over network gaps, to optimize the connectivity of the semantic network. In ConceptNet 2, a new system for weighting knowledge was implemented, which scores each binary assertion based on how many times it was uttered in the OMCS corpus, and on how well it can be inferred indirectly from other facts in ConceptNet. In ConceptNet 3 [47], users can also participate in the process of refining knowledge by evaluating existing statements on Open Mind Commons [97], the new interface for collecting commonsense knowledge from users over the Web.

By giving the user many forms of feedback and using inferences by analogy to find appropriate questions to ask, Open Mind Commons can learn well-connected structures of commonsense knowledge, refine its existing knowledge, and build analogies that lead to even more powerful inferences. ConceptNet 4 includes data that was imported from the online game Verbosity. It also includes the initial import of the Chinese ConceptNet. ConceptNet 5 [98], eventually, contains knowledge from English Wikipedia, specifically from DBPedia, which extracts knowledge from the info-boxes that appear on articles, and ReVerb, a machine-reading project extracting relational knowledge from the actual text of each article. It also includes a large amount of content from the English Wiktionary, including synonyms, antonyms, translations of concepts into hundreds of languages, and multiple labelled word senses for many English words.

ConceptNet 5 contains more dictionary-style knowledge coming from WordNet and some knowledge about people's intuitive word associations coming from

GWAPs. Previous versions of ConceptNet have been distributed as idiosyncratic database structures plus some software to interact with them. ConceptNet 5 is not a piece of software or a database, but a hypergraph, that is, a graph that has edges about edges. Each statement in ConceptNet, in fact, has justifications pointing to it, explaining where it comes from and how reliable the information seems to be. ConceptNet is a good source of commonsense knowledge but alone is not enough for sentiment analysis tasks as it specifies how concepts are semantically related to each other but often lacks connections between concepts that convey the same kind of emotion or similar polarity. To overcome such a hurdle, affective knowledge from WNA is added.

3.2.2 AffectNet Matrix

In Chinese culture (and many others), the concepts of 'heart' and 'mind' used to be expressed by the same word as it was believed that consciousness and thoughts came from the cardiac muscle. In human cognition, in fact, thinking and feeling are mutually present: emotions are often the product of our thoughts, as well as our reflections are often the product of our affective states. Emotions are intrinsically part of our mental activity and play a key role in communication and decision-making processes. Emotion is a chain of events made up of feedback loops. Feelings and behavior can affect cognition, just as cognition can influence feeling. Emotion, cognition, and action interact in feedback loops and emotion can be viewed in a structural model tied to adaptation [88].

There is actually no fundamental opposition between emotion and reason. In fact, it may be argued that reason consists of basing choices on the perspectives of emotions at some later time. Reason dictates not giving in to one's impulses because doing so may cause greater suffering later [43]. Reason does not necessarily imply exertion of the voluntary capacities to suppress emotion. It does not necessarily involve depriving certain aspects of reality of their emotive powers.

On the contrary, our voluntary capacities allow us to draw more of reality into the sphere of emotion. They allow one's emotions to be elicited not merely by the proximal, or the perceptual, or that which directly interferes with one's actions, but by that which, in fact, touches on one's concerns, whether proximal or distal, whether occurring now or in the future, whether interfering with one's own life or that of others. Cognitive functions serve emotions and biological needs. Information from the environment is evaluated in terms of its ability to satisfy or frustrate needs. What is particularly significant is that each new cognitive experience that is biologically important is connected with an emotional reaction such as fear, pleasure, pain, disgust, or depression [81].

I order to build a semantic network that contains both semantic and affective knowledge, ConceptNet and WNA are blended together by combining the matrix representations of the two knowledge bases linearly into a single matrix, in which the information between the two initial sources is shared. The first step to create the affective blend is to transform the input data so that it can all be represented in the same matrix. To do this, the lemma forms of ConceptNet concepts are aligned with the lemma forms of the words in WNA and the most common relations in the affective knowledge base are mapped into ConceptNet's set of relations, e.g., Hypernym into *IsA* and Holonym into *PartOf*. In particular, ConceptNet is first converted into a matrix by dividing each assertion into two parts: a concept and a feature, where a feature is simply the assertion with the first or the second concept left unspecified such as 'a wheel is part of' or 'is a kind of liquid'. The entries in the resulting matrix are positive or negative numbers, depending on the reliability of the assertions, and their magnitude increases logarithmically with the confidence score. WNA, similarly, is represented as a matrix where rows are affective concepts and columns are features related to these.

The result of aligning the matrix representations of ConceptNet and WNA is a new affective semantic network, in which commonsense concepts are linked to a hierarchy of affective domain labels. In such a semantic network, termed AffectNet,[6] commonsense and affective knowledge are in fact combined, not just concomitant, i.e., everyday life concepts like 'have breakfast', 'meet people', or 'watch tv' are linked to affective domain labels like 'joy', 'anger', or 'surprise'. Because the AffectNet graph is made of triples of the format <concept-relationship-concept>, the entire knowledge repository can be visualized as a large matrix, with every known concept of some statement being a row and every known semantic feature (relationship + concept) being a column. Such a representation has several advantages including the possibility to perform cumulative analogy [33, 104]. Cumulative analogy is performed by first selecting a set of nearest neighbors, in terms of similarity, of the input concept and then by projecting known properties of this set onto not known properties of the concept (Table 3.4).

It is inherent to human nature to try to categorize things and people, finding patterns and forms they have in common. One of the most intuitive ways to relate two entities is through their similarity. Similarity is one of the six Gestalt principles which guide the human perception of the world, the remaining ones being: Proximity, Closure, Good Continuation, Common Fate, and Good Form. According to Merriam Webster, 'similarity' is a quality that makes one person or thing like another and 'similar' means having characteristics in common. There are many ways in which objects can be perceived as similar, such as having similar color, shape, size, and texture. If we move away from mere visual stimuli, we can apply the same principles to define a similarity between concepts based on shared semantic features. For AffectNet, however, such a process is rather time- and resource-consuming as its matrix representation is made of several thousands columns (fat matrix). In order to perform analogical reasoning in a faster and more efficient manner, such a matrix can be represented as a vector space by applying multi-dimensionality reduction techniques that decrease the number of semantic features associated with each concept without compromising too much knowledge representation.

---

[6]http://sentic.net/affectnet.zip

Table 3.4 Cumulative analogy allows for the inference of new pieces of knowledge by comparing similar concepts. In the example, it is inferred that the concept `special_occasion` causes joy as it shares the same set of semantic features with `wedding` and `birthday` (which also cause joy) (Source: The Authors)

Concepts		Semantic Features (relationship+concept)				
	...	*Causes* joy	*IsA* event	*UsedFor* housework	*MotivatedBy* celebration	...
⋮		⋮	⋮	⋮	⋮	
wedding	...	x	x	−	x	...
broom	...	−	−	x	−	...
special_occasion	...	**x?**	x	−	x	...
birthday	...	x	x	−	x	...
⋮		⋮	⋮	⋮	⋮	

3.2.3 AffectiveSpace

The best way to solve a problem is to already know a solution for it. However, if we have to face a problem we have never met before, we need to use our intuition. Intuition can be explained as the process of making analogies between the current problem and the ones solved in the past to find a suitable solution. Marvin Minsky attributes this property to the so called 'difference-engines' [77]. This particular kind of agents operates by recognizing differences between the current state and the desired state, and acting to reduce each difference by invoking K-lines that turn on suitable solution methods.

This kind of thinking is maybe the essence of our supreme intelligence since in everyday life no two situations are ever the same and have to perform this action continuously. To emulate such a process, AffectiveSpace[7] [19], a novel affective commonsense knowledge visualization and analysis system, is used. The human mind constructs intelligible meanings by continuously compressing over vital relations [41]. The compression principles aim to transform diffuse and distended conceptual structures to more focused versions so as to become more congenial for human understanding. To this end, principal component analysis (PCA) has been applied on the matrix representation of AffectNet.

In particular, truncated singular value decomposition (TSVD) has been preferred to other dimensionality reduction techniques for its simplicity, relatively low computational cost, and compactness. TSVD, in fact, is particularly suitable for measuring the cross-correlations between affective commonsense concepts as it uses an orthogonal transformation to convert the set of possibly correlated commonsense features associated with each concept into a set of values of uncorrelated variables

---

[7]http://sentic.net/affectivespace.zip

(the principal components of the SVD). By using Lanczos' method [60], moreover, the generalization process is relatively fast (a few seconds), despite the size and the sparseness of AffectNet. The objective of such compression is to allow many details in the blend of ConceptNet and WNA to be removed such that the blend only consists of a few essential features that represent the global picture. Applying TSVD on AffectNet, in fact, causes it to describe other features that could apply to known affective concepts by analogy: if a concept in the matrix has no value specified for a feature owned by many similar concepts, then by analogy the concept is likely to have that feature as well. In other words, concepts and features that point in similar directions and, therefore, have high dot products, are good candidates for analogies.

A pioneering work on understanding and visualizing the affective information associated with natural language text was conducted by Osgood et al. [84]. Osgood used multi-dimensional scaling (MDS) to create visualizations of affective words based on similarity ratings of the words provided to subjects from different cultures. Words can be thought of as points in a multi-dimensional space and the similarity ratings represent the distances between these words. MDS projects these distances to points in a smaller dimensional space (usually two or three dimensions). Similarly, AffectiveSpace aims to grasp the semantic and affective similarity between different concepts by plotting them into a multi-dimensional vector space [24]. Unlike Osgood's space, however, the building blocks of AffectiveSpace are not simply a limited set of similarity ratings between affect words, but rather millions of confidence scores related to pieces of commonsense knowledge linked to a hierarchy of affective domain labels. Rather than merely determined by a few human annotators and represented as a word-word matrix, in fact, AffectiveSpace is built upon an affective commonsense knowledge base, namely AffectNet, represented as a concept-feature matrix. After performing TSVD on such matrix, hereby termed A for the sake of conciseness, a low-rank approximation of it is obtained, that is, a new matrix $\tilde{A} = U_k \Sigma_k V_k^T$.

This approximation is based on minimizing the Frobenius norm of the difference between A and $\tilde{A}$ under the constraint $rank(\tilde{A}) = k$. For the Eckart–Young theorem [39], it represents the best approximation of A in the least-square sense, in fact:

$$\min_{\tilde{A}|rank(\tilde{A})=k} |A - \tilde{A}| = \min_{\tilde{A}|rank(\tilde{A})=k} |\Sigma - U^*\tilde{A}V| = \min_{\tilde{A}|rank(\tilde{A})=k} |\Sigma - S| \qquad (3.1)$$

assuming that $\tilde{A}$ has the form $\tilde{A} = USV^*$, where S is diagonal. From the rank constraint, i.e., S has k non-zero diagonal entries, the minimum of the above statement is obtained as follows:

$$\min_{\tilde{A}|rank(\tilde{A})=k} |\Sigma - S| = \min_{s_i} \sqrt{\sum_{i=1}^{n} (\sigma_i - s_i)^2} \qquad (3.2)$$

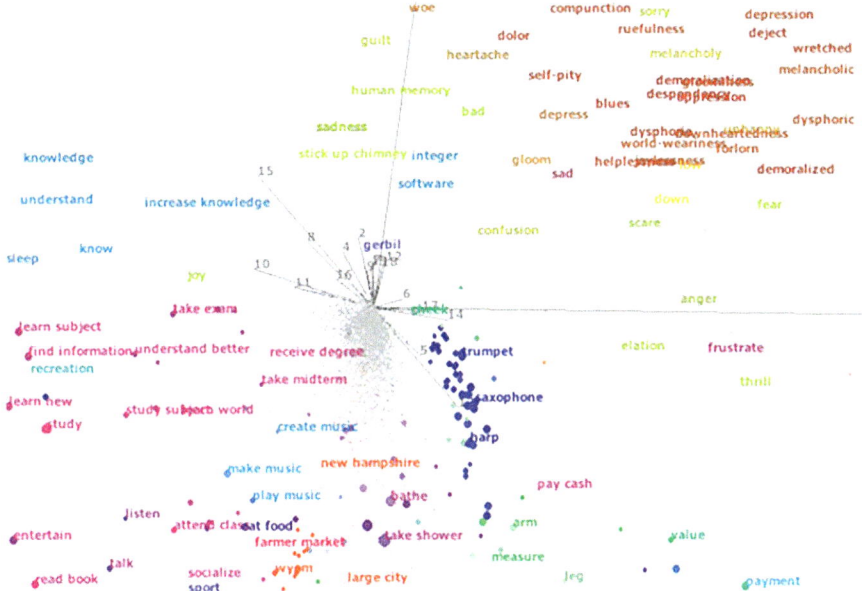

Fig. 3.13 A sketch of AffectiveSpace. Affectively positive concepts (in the bottom-left corner) and affectively negative concepts (in the up-right corner) are floating in the multi-dimensional vector space (Source: [19])

$$\min_{s_i} \sqrt{\sum_{i=1}^{n} (\sigma_i - s_i)^2} = \min_{s_i} \sqrt{\sum_{i=1}^{k} (\sigma_i - s_i)^2 + \sum_{i=k+1}^{n} \sigma_i^2} = \sqrt{\sum_{i=k+1}^{n} \sigma_i^2} \qquad (3.3)$$

Therefore, $\tilde{A}$ of rank k is the best approximation of A in the Frobenius norm sense when $\sigma_i = s_i$ $(i = 1, \dots, k)$ and the corresponding singular vectors are the same as those of A. If all but the first k principal components are discarded, commonsense concepts and emotions are represented by vectors of k coordinates. These coordinates can be seen as describing concepts in terms of 'eigenmoods' that form the axes of AffectiveSpace, i.e., the basis $e_0, \dots, e_{k-1}$ of the vector space (Fig. 3.13). For example, the most significant eigenmood, e_0, represents concepts with positive affective valence. That is, the larger a concept's component in the e_0 direction is, the more affectively positive it is likely to be.

Concepts with negative e_0 components, then, are likely to have negative affective valence. Thus, by exploiting the information sharing property of TSVD, concepts with the same affective valence are likely to have similar features – that is, concepts conveying the same emotion tend to fall near each other in AffectiveSpace. Concept similarity does not depend on their absolute positions in the vector space, but rather on the angle they make with the origin. For example concepts such as 'beautiful day', 'birthday party', and 'make person happy' are found very close in direction in the vector space, while concepts like 'feel guilty', 'be laid off', and 'shed tear' are found in a completely different direction (nearly opposite with respect to the centre of the space).

The problem with this kind of representation is that it is not scalable: when the number of concepts and of semantic features grows, the AffectNet matrix becomes too high-dimensional and too sparse for SVD to be computed [9]. Although there has been a body of research on seeking for fast approximations of the SVD, the approximate methods are at most ≈ 5 times faster than the standard one [76], making it not attractive for real-world big data applications. It has been conjectured that there might be simple but powerful meta-algorithms underlying neuronal learning [64].

These meta-algorithms should be fast, scalable, effective, with few-to-no specific assumptions, and biologically plausible [9]. Optimizing all the $\approx 10^{15}$ connections through the last few million years' evolution is very unlikely [9]. Alternatively, nature probably only optimizes the global connectivity (mainly the white matter), but leaves the other details to randomness [9]. In order to cope with the ever-growing number of concepts and semantic features, thus, SVD is replaced with random projection (RP) [12], a data-oblivious method, to map the original high-dimensional data-set into a much lower-dimensional subspace by using a Gaussian $N(0, 1)$ matrix, while preserving the pair-wise distances with high probability. This theoretically solid and empirically verified statement follows Johnson Lindenstrauss (JL) Lemma [9]. The JL Lemma states that with high probability, for all pairs of points $x, y \in X$ simultaneously

$$\sqrt{\frac{m}{d}} \parallel x - y \parallel_2 (1 - \varepsilon) \leq \parallel \Phi x - \Phi y \parallel_2 \leq \qquad (3.4)$$

$$\leq \sqrt{\frac{m}{d}} \parallel x - y \parallel_2 (1 + \varepsilon), \qquad (3.5)$$

where X is a set of vectors in Euclidean space, d is the original dimension of this Euclidean space, m is the dimension of the space we wish to reduce the data points to, ε is a tolerance parameter measuring to what extent is the maximum allowed distortion rate of the metric space, and Φ is a random matrix.

Structured random projection for making matrix multiplication much faster was introduced in [92]. Achlioptas [1] proposed *sparse random projection* to replace the Gaussian matrix with i.i.d. entries in

$$\phi_{ji} = \sqrt{s} \begin{cases} 1 & \text{with prob. } \frac{1}{2s} \\ 0 & \text{with prob. } 1 - \frac{1}{s}, \\ -1 & \text{with prob. } \frac{1}{2s} \end{cases} \qquad (3.6)$$

where one can achieve a ×3 speedup by setting $s = 3$, since only $\frac{1}{3}$ of the data need to be processed. However, since AffectNet is already too sparse, using sparse random projection is not advisable.

When the number of features is much larger than the number of training samples ($d \gg n$), subsampled randomized Hadamard transform (SRHT) is preferred, as it behaves very much like Gaussian random matrices but accelerates the process from $\mathcal{O}(nd)$ to $\mathcal{O}(n \log d)$ time [70]. Following [70, 103], for $d = 2^p$ where p is any positive integer, a SRHT can be defined as:

$$\Phi = \sqrt{\frac{d}{m}} \text{RHD} \tag{3.7}$$

where

- m is the number we want to subsample from d features randomly.
- R is a random $m \times d$ matrix. The rows of R are m uniform samples (without replacement) from the standard basis of $\mathbb{R}^d$.
- $H \in \mathbb{R}^{d \times d}$ is a normalized Walsh-Hadamard matrix, which is defined recursively: $H_d = \begin{bmatrix} H_{d/2} & H_{d/2} \\ H_{d/2} & H_{d/2} \end{bmatrix}$ with $H_2 = \begin{bmatrix} +1 & +1 \\ +1 & -1 \end{bmatrix}$.
- D is a $d \times d$ diagonal matrix and the diagonal elements are i.i.d. Rademacher random variables.

The subsequent analysis only relies on the distances and angles between pairs of vectors (i.e., the Euclidean geometry information), and it is sufficient to set the projected space to be logarithmic in the size of the data [8] and apply SRHT.

The key to perform commonsense reasoning is to find a good trade-off for representing knowledge. Since in life two situations are never exactly the same, no representation should be too concrete, or it will not apply to new situations, but, at the same time, no representation should be too abstract, or it will suppress too many details. AffectNet already supports different representations, in fact, it maintains different ways of conveying the same idea with redundant concepts, e.g., 'car' and 'automobile', that can be reconciled through background linguistic knowledge, if necessary. Within AffectiveSpace, this knowledge representation trade-off can be seen in the choice of the vector space dimensionality (Table 3.5).

The number k of singular values selected to build AffectiveSpace is a measure of the trade-off between precision and efficiency in the representation of the affective commonsense knowledge base. The bigger k is, the more precisely AffectiveSpace represents AffectNet's knowledge, but generating the vector space is slower, and so is computing dot products between concepts. The smaller k is, on the other hand, the more efficiently AffectiveSpace represents affective commonsense knowledge both in terms of vector space generation and of dot product computation. However, too few dimensions risk not to correctly represent AffectNet as concepts defined with too few features tend to be too close to each other in the vector space and, hence, not easily distinguishable and clusterable.

Table 3.5 Some examples of LiveJournal posts where affective information is not conveyed explicitly through affect words (Source: [22])

Mood	LiveJournal posts	Concepts
Happy	Finally I got my student cap ! I am officially high school graduate now ! Our dog Tanja, me, Timo (our art teacher) and EmmaMe, Tanja, Emma and Tiia Only two weeks to Japan!!	Student; School graduate; Japan
Happy	I got a kitten as an early birthday gift on Monday. Abby was smelly, dirty, and knawing on the metal bars of the kitten carrier though somewhat calm when I picked her up. We took her. She threw up on me on the ride home and repeatedly keeps sneesing in my face	Kitten; Birthday gift; Metal bar; Face
Sad	Hi. Can I ask a favor from you? This will only take a minute. Please pray for Marie, my friends' dog a labrador, for she has canine distemper. Her lower half is paralysed and she's having locked jaw. My friends' family is feeding her through syringe	Friends; Dog; Labrador; Canine distemper; Jaw; Syringe
Sad	My uncle paul passed away on february 16, 2008. He lost his battle with cancer. I remember spending time with him and my aunt nina when they babysat me. We would go to taco bell to eat nachos	Uncle; Battle; Cancer; Aunt; Taco bell; Nachos

In order to find a good k, AffectiveSpace was tested on a benchmark for affective commonsense knowledge (BACK) built by applying CF-IOF (concept frequency – inverse opinion frequency) [23] on the 5,000 posts of the LiveJournal corpus. CF-IOF is a technique that identifies common domain-dependent semantics in order to evaluate how important a concept is to a set of opinions concerning the same topic. Firstly, the frequency of a concept c for a given domain d is calculated by counting the occurrences of the concept c in the set of available d-tagged opinions and dividing the result by the sum of number of occurrences of all concepts in the set of opinions concerning d. This frequency is then multiplied by the logarithm of the inverse frequency of the concept in the whole collection of opinions, that is:

$$CF\text{-}IOF_{c,d} = \frac{n_{c,d}}{\sum_k n_{k,d}} \log \sum_k \frac{n_k}{n_c} \tag{3.8}$$

where $n_{c,d}$ is the number of occurrences of concept c in the set of opinions tagged as d, n_k is the total number of concept occurrences, and n_c is the number of occurrences of c in the whole set of opinions.

A high weight in CF-IOF is reached by a high concept frequency in a given domain and a low frequency of the concept in the whole collection of opinions. Specifically, CF-IOF weighting was exploited to filter out common concepts in the LiveJournal corpus and to detect relevant mood-dependent semantics for the set of 24 emotions defined by Plutchik [88]. The result was a benchmark of 2,000 affective concepts that were screened by 21 English-speaking students who were asked to map each concept to the 24 different emotional categories, which form the Hourglass of Emotions [25] (explained later). Results obtained were averaged (Table 3.6). BACK's concepts were compared with the classification results obtained by applying the AffectiveSpace process using different values of

Table 3.6 Distribution of concepts through the Pleasantness dimension. The affective information associated with most concepts concentrates around the centre of the Hourglass, rather than its extremes (Source: [22])

Level	Label	Frequency (%)
G(−1)	Grief	14.3
G(−2/3)	Sadness	19.8
G(−1/3)	Pensiveness	11.4
0	Neutral	10.5
G(1/3)	Serenity	20.6
G(2/3)	Joy	18.3
G(1)	Ecstasy	5.1

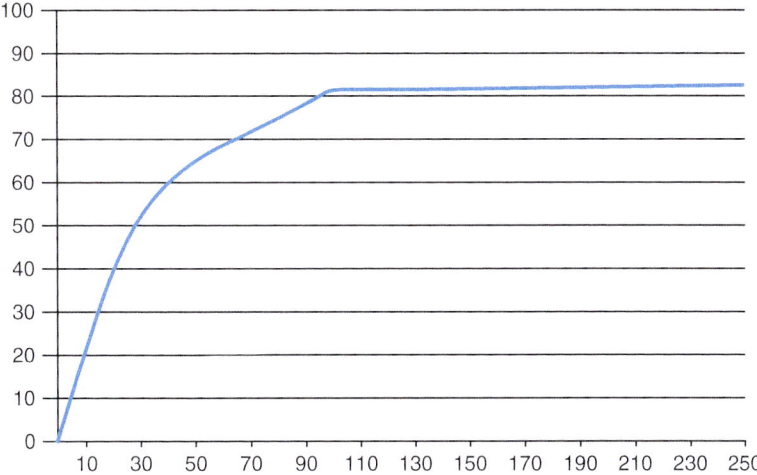

Fig. 3.14 Accuracy values achieved by testing AffectiveSpace on BACK, with dimensionality spanning from 1 to 250. The best trade-off between precision and efficiency is obtained around 100 (Source: [22])

k, from 1 to 250. As shown in Fig. 3.14, the best trade-off is achieved at 100, as selecting more than 100 singular values does not improve accuracy significantly.

The distribution of the values of each AffectiveSpace dimension is bell-shaped, with different centers and different degree of dispersion around them. Affective commonsense concepts, in fact, tend to be close to the origin of the vector space (Fig. 3.15). In order to more uniformly distribute concept density in AffectiveSpace, an alternative strategy to represent the vector space was investigated. Such strategy consists in centering the values of the distribution of each dimension on the origin and in mapping dimensions according to a transformation $x \in \mathbb{R} \mapsto x^* \in [−1, 1]$. This transformation is often pivotal for better clustering AffectiveSpace as the vector space tends to have different grades of dispersion of data points across different dimensions, with some space regions more densely populated than others.

The switch to a different space configuration helps to distribute data more uniformly, possibly leading to an improved (or, at least, different) reasoning process. In particular, the transformation $x_{ij} \mapsto x_{ij} − \mu_i$ is first applied, being μ_i the average

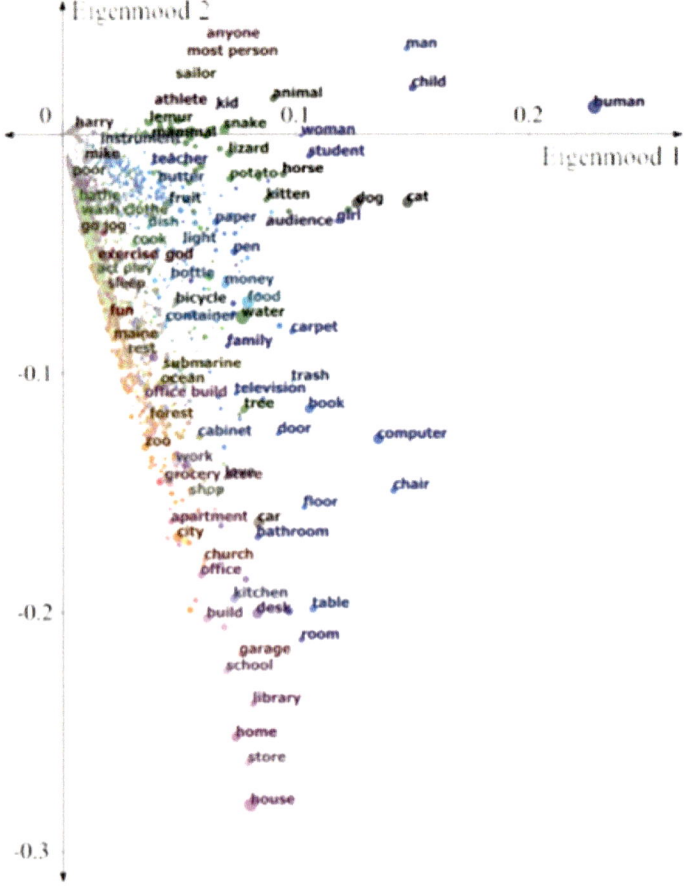

Fig. 3.15 A two-dimensional projection (first and second eigenmoods) of AffectiveSpace. From this visualization, it is evident that concept density is usually higher near the centre of the space (Source: [22])

of all values of the i-th dimension. Then a normalization is applied, combining the previous transformation with a new one $x_{ij} \mapsto \frac{x_{ij}}{a \cdot \sigma_i}$, where σ_i is the standard deviation calculated on the i-th dimension and a is a coefficient that can modify the same proportion of data that is represented within a specified interval.

Finally, in order to ensure that all components of the vectors in the defined space are within $[-1, 1]$ (i.e., that the Chebyshev distance between the origin and each vector is smaller or equal to 1), a final transformation $x_{ij} \mapsto s(x_{ij})$ is needed, where $s(x)$ is a sigmoid function. Different choices for the sigmoid function may be made, influencing how 'fast' the function approaches the unit value while the independent variable approaches infinity. Combining the proposed transformations, two possible mapping functions are expressed in the following formulae (3.9) and (3.10):

$$x_{ij}^* = tanh\left(\frac{x_{ij} - \mu_i}{a \cdot \sigma_i}\right) \tag{3.9}$$

$$x_{ij}^* = \frac{x_{ij} - \mu_i}{a \cdot \sigma_i + \left|x_{ij} - \mu_i\right|} \tag{3.10}$$

This space transformation leads to two main advantages, which could be of notable importance depending on the problem being tackled. Firstly, this different space configuration ensures that each dimension is equally important by avoiding that the information provided by dimensions with higher (i.e., more distant from the origin) averages predominates. Secondly, normalizing according to the standard deviations of each dimension allows for a more uniform distribution of data around the origin, leading to a full use of information potential.

3.3 Knowledge-Based Reasoning

This section describes the techniques adopted for generating semantics and sentics from the three different commonsense knowledge representations described above. In particular, semantics are inferred by means of spreading activation (Sect. 3.3.1) while sentics are created through the ensemble application of an emotion categorization model (Sect. 3.3.2) and a set of neural networks (Sect. 3.3.3).

3.3.1 Sentic Activation

An important difference between traditional AI systems and human intelligence is our ability to harness commonsense knowledge gleaned from a lifetime of learning and experiences to inform our decision-making and behavior.

This allows humans to adapt easily to novel situations where AI fails catastrophically for lack of situation-specific rules and generalization capabilities. In order for machines to exploit commonsense knowledge in reasoning as humans do, moreover, we need to endow them with human-like reasoning strategies. In problem-solving situations, in particular, several analogous representations of the same problem should be maintained in parallel while trying to solve it so that, when problem-solving begins to fail while using one representation, the system can switch to one of the others [28].

Sentic activation [27] is a two-level reasoning framework for the generation of semantics (Fig. 3.16). By representing commonsense knowledge redundantly at three levels (semantic network, matrix, and vector space), sentic activation implements a reasoning loop that solves the problem of relevance in spreading activation by guiding the activation of nodes through analogical reasoning. In particular, the

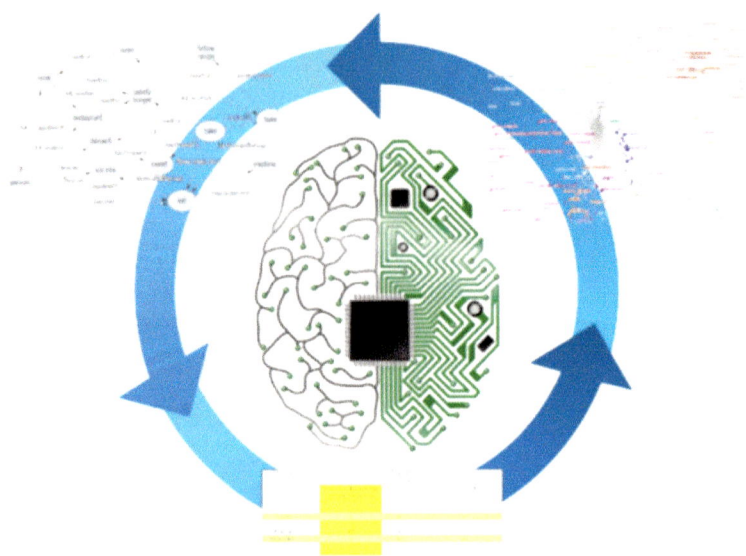

Fig. 3.16 The sentic activation loop. Commonsense knowledge is represented redundantly at three levels (semantic network, matrix, and vector space) in order to solve the problem of relevance in spreading activation (Source: Sentic computing [22])

framework limits the activation of concepts in AffectNet by exploiting the set of semantically related concepts generated by AffectiveSpace.

Sentic activation is inspired by the current thinking in cognitive psychology, which suggests that humans process information at a minimum of two distinct levels. There is extensive evidence for the existence of two (or more) processing systems within the human brain, one that involves fast, parallel, unconscious processing, and one that involves slow, serial, more conscious processing [32, 40, 57, 95]. Dual-process models of automatic and controlled social cognition have been proposed in nearly every domain of social psychology. Evidence from neurosciences supports this separation, with identifiably different brain regions involved in each of the two systems [68].

Such systems, termed U-level (unconscious) and C-level (conscious), can operate simultaneously or sequentially, and are most effective in different contexts. The former, in particular, works intuitively, effortlessly, globally, and emotionally (Sect. 3.3.1.1). The latter, in turn, works logically, systematically, effortfully, and rationally (Sect. 3.3.1.2).

3.3.1.1   Unconscious Reasoning

In recent years, neuroscience has contributed a lot to the study of emotions through the development of novel methods for studying emotional processes and their neural correlates. In particular, new methods used in affective neuroscience, e.g., functional magnetic resonance imaging (FMRI), lesion studies, genetics, electro-physiology, paved the way towards the understanding of the neural circuitry that underlies emotional experience and of the manner in which emotional states influence health and life outcomes. A key contribution in the last two decades has been to provide evidence against the notion that emotions are subcortical and limbic, whereas cognition is cortical.

This notion was reinforcing the flawed Cartesian dichotomy between thoughts and feelings [38]. There is now ample evidence that the neural substrates of cognition and emotion overlap substantially [37]. Cognitive processes, such as memory encoding and retrieval, causal reasoning, deliberation, goal appraisal, and planning, operate continually throughout the experience of emotion. This evidence points to the importance of considering the affective components of any human-computer interaction [18]. Affective neuroscience, in particular, has provided evidence that elements of emotional learning can occur without awareness [82] and elements of emotional behavior do not require explicit processing [17]. Affective information processing, in fact, mainly takes place at unconscious level (U-level) [40].

Reasoning, at this level, relies on experience and intuition, which allow for fast and effortless problem-solving. Hence, rather than reflecting upon various considerations in sequence, the U-level forms a global impression of the different issues. In addition, rather than applying logical rules or symbolic codes (e.g., words or numbers), the U-level considers vivid representations of objects or events. Such representations are laden with the emotions, details, features, and sensations that correspond to the objects or events.

Such human capability of summarizing the huge amount of inputs and outputs of previous situations, in order to find useful patterns that might work at the present time, is hereby implemented by means of AffectiveSpace. By reducing the dimensionality of the matrix representation of AffectNet, in fact, AffectiveSpace compresses the feature space of affective commonsense knowledge into one that allows for better global insight and human-scale understanding. In cognitive science, the term 'compression' refers to transforming diffuse and distended conceptual structures that are less congenial to human understanding so that they become better suited to our human-scale ways of thinking.

Compression is hereby achieved by balancing the number of singular values discarded when synthesizing AffectiveSpace, in a way that the affective commonsense knowledge representation is neither too concrete nor too abstract with respect to the detail granularity needed for performing a particular task. The reasoning-by-analogy capabilities of AffectiveSpace, hence, are exploited at U-level to achieve digital intuition about the input data. In particular, the vector space representation of affective commonsense knowledge is clustered according the Hourglass model using the sentic medoids technique [26], in a way that concepts that are semantically and affectively related to the input data can be intuitively retrieved by analogy and unconsciously crop out to the C-level.

3.3.1.2 Conscious Reasoning

U-level and C-level are two conceptual systems that operate by different rules of
inference. While the former operates emotionally and intuitively, the latter relies
on logic and rationality. In particular, the C-level analyzes issues with effort, logic,
and deliberation rather than relying on intuition. Hence, while at U-level the vector
space representation of AffecNet is exploited to intuitively guess semantic and
affective relations between concepts, at C-level associations between concepts are
made according to the actual connections between different nodes in the graph
representation of affective commonsense knowledge.

Memory is not a 'thing' that is stored somewhere in a mental warehouse and can
be pulled out and brought to the fore. Rather, it is a potential for reactivation of a
set of concepts that together constitute a particular meaning. Associative memory
involves the unconscious activation of networks of association–thoughts, feelings,
wishes, fears, and perceptions that are connected, so that activation of one node in
the network leads to activation of the others [106].

Sentic activation aims to implement such a process through the ensemble
application of multi-dimensionality reduction and graph mining techniques. Specifically, the semantically and affectively related concepts retrieved by means of
AffectiveSpace at U-level are fed into AffectNet in order to crawl it according to
how such seed concepts are interconnected to each other and to other concepts in
the semantic network. To this end, spectral association [48] is employed. Spectral
association is a technique that assigns values, or activations, to seed concepts and
spreads their values across the AffectNet graph.

This operation, which is an approximation of many steps of spreading activation,
transfers the most activation to concepts that are connected to the seed concepts by
short paths or many different paths in affective commonsense knowledge. These
related concepts are likely to have similar affective values. This can be seen as
an alternate way of assigning affective values to all concepts, which simplifies the
process by not relying on an outside resource such as WNA. In particular, a matrix
A that relates concepts to other concepts, instead of their features, is built and the
scores are added up over all relations that relate one concept to another, disregarding
direction.

Applying A to a vector containing a single concept spreads that concept's value
to its connected concepts. Applying A^2 spreads that value to concepts connected
by two links (including back to the concept itself). But the desired operation is to
spread the activation through any number of links, with diminishing returns, so the
operator wanted is:

$$1 + A + \frac{A^2}{2!} + \frac{A^3}{3!} + \ldots = e^A \qquad (3.11)$$

This odd operator, e^A, can be calculated because A can be factored. A is already
symmetric, so instead of applying Lanczos' method [60] to AA^T and getting
the SVD, it can be applied directly to A to obtain the spectral decomposition

$A = V \Lambda V^T$. As before, this expression can be raised to any power and everything but the power of Λ cancelled. Therefore, $e^A = Ve^\Lambda V^T$. This simple twist on the SVD allows for the calculation of calculate spreading activation over the whole matrix instantly. As with the SVD, these matrices can be truncated to k axes and, therefore, space can be saved while generalizing from similar concepts. The matrix can also be rescaled so that activation values have a maximum of 1 and do not tend to collect in highly-connected concepts such as 'person', by normalizing the truncated rows of $Ve^{\Lambda/2}$ to unit vectors, and multiplying that matrix by its transpose to get a rescaled version of $Ve^\Lambda V^T$. Spectral association can spread not only positive, but also negative activation values. Hence, unconscious reasoning at U-level is exploited not only to retrieve concepts that are most semantically and affectively related, but also concepts that are most likely to be unrelated with the input data (lowest dot product).

While the former are exploited to spread semantics and sentics across the AffectNet graph, the latter are used to contain such an activation in a way that potentially unrelated concepts (and their twins) do not get triggered. This brain-inspired ensemble application of dimensionality reduction and graph mining techniques (hereby referred as unconscious and conscious reasoning, respectively) allows sentic activation to more efficiently infer semantics and sentics from natural language text.

Sentic activation was tested on the benchmark for affective commonsense knowledge (BACK) by comparing concept classification results obtained by applying the AffectiveSpace process (U-level), spectral association (C-level), and the ensemble of U-level and C-level. Results showed that sentic activation achieves +13.9% and +8.2% accuracy than the AffectiveSpace process and spectral association, respectively.

3.3.2 *Hourglass Model*

The study of emotions is one of the most confused (and still open) chapters in the history of psychology. This is mainly due to the ambiguity of natural language, which does not facilitate the description of mixed emotions in an unequivocal way. Love and other emotional words like anger and fear, in fact, are suitcase words (many different meanings packed in), not clearly defined and meaning different things to different people [78].

Hence, more than 90 definitions of emotions have been offered over the past century and there are almost as many theories of emotion, not to mention a complex array of overlapping words in our languages to describe them. Some categorizations include cognitive versus non-cognitive emotions, instinctual (from the amygdala) versus cognitive (from the prefrontal cortex) emotions, and also categorizations based on duration, as some emotions occur over a period of seconds (e.g., surprise), whereas others can last years (e.g., love).

The James-Lange theory posits that emotional experience is largely due to the experience of bodily changes [56]. Its main contribution is the emphasis it places on the embodiment of emotions, especially the argument that changes in the bodily concomitants of emotions can alter their experienced intensity. Most contemporary neuroscientists endorse a modified James-Lange view, in which bodily feedback modulates the experience of emotion [36]. In this view, emotions are related to certain activities in brain areas that direct our attention, motivate our behavior, and determine the significance of what is going on around us.

Pioneering works by Broca [15], Papez [86], and MacLean [72] suggested that emotion is related to a group of structures in the centre of the brain called limbic system (or paleomammalian brain), which includes the hypothalamus, cingulate cortex, hippocampi, and other structures. More recent research, however, has shown that some of these limbic structures are not as directly related to emotion as others are, while some non-limbic structures have been found to be of greater emotional relevance [63].

In [88] model, the vertical dimension represents intensity and the radial dimension represents degrees of similarity among the emotions. Besides bi-dimensional approaches, a commonly used set for emotion dimension is the <arousal, valence, dominance> set, which is known in the literature also by different names, including <evaluation, activation, power> and <pleasure, arousal, dominance> [75]. Recent evidence suggests there should be a fourth dimension: Fontaine et al., reported consistent results from various cultures where a set of four dimensions is found in user studies, namely <valence, potency, arousal, unpredictability> [42]. Dimensional representations of affect are attractive mainly because they provide a way of describing emotional states that is more tractable than using words. This is of particular importance when dealing with naturalistic data, where a wide range of emotional states occurs. Similarly, they are much more able to deal with non-discrete emotions and variations in emotional states over time [34], since in such cases changing from one universal emotion label to another would not make much sense in real life scenarios. Dimensional approaches, however, have a few limitations. Although the dimensional space allows to compare affect words according to their reciprocal distance, it usually does not allow making operations between these, e.g., for studying compound emotions. Most dimensional representations, moreover, do not model the fact that two or more emotions may be experienced at the same time. Eventually, all such approaches work at word level, which makes them unable to grasp the affective valence of multiple-word concepts.

The Hourglass of Emotions [25] is an affective categorization model inspired by Plutchik's studies on human emotions [88]. It reinterprets Plutchik's model by organizing primary emotions around four independent but concomitant dimensions, whose different levels of activation make up the total emotional state of the mind. Such a reinterpretation is inspired by Minsky's theory of the mind, according to which brain activity consists of different independent resources and that emotional states result from turning some set of these resources on and turning another set of them off [78]. This way, the model can potentially synthesize the full range of emotional experiences in terms of Pleasantness, Attention, Sensitivity, and Aptitude, as the different combined values of the four affective dimensions can also model affective states we do not have a specific name for, due to the ambiguity of natural language and the elusive nature of emotions.

The main motivation for the design of the model is the concept-level inference of the cognitive and affective information associated with text. Such faceted information is needed, within sentic computing, for a feature-based sentiment analysis, where the affective commonsense knowledge associated with natural language opinions has to be objectively assessed. Therefore, the Hourglass model systematically excludes what are variously known as self-conscious or moral emotions, e.g., pride, guilt, shame, embarrassment, moral outrage, or humiliation [62, 66, 93, 102]. Such emotions, in fact, present a blind spot for models rooted in basic emotions, because they are by definition contingent on subjective moral standards. The distinction between guilt and shame, for example, is based in the attribution of negativity to the self or to the act. Hence, guilt arises when believing to have done a bad thing, and shame arises when thinking to be a bad person.

This matters because, in turn, these emotions have been shown to have different consequences in terms of action tendencies. Likewise, an emotion such as *schaden-freude* is essentially a form of pleasure, but it is crucially different from pride or happiness because of the object of the emotion (the misfortune of another that is not caused by the self), and the resulting action tendency (do not express).

However, since the Hourglass model currently focuses on the objective inference of affective information associated with natural language opinions, appraisal-based emotions are not taken into account within the present version of the model. The Hourglass model (Fig. 3.17) is a biologically-inspired and psychologically-motivated model based on the idea that emotional states result from the selective activation/disactivation of different resources in the brain. Each such selection changes how we think by changing our brain's activities: the state of anger, for example, appears to select a set of resources that help us react with more speed and strength while also suppressing some other resources that usually make us act prudently.

Evidence of this theory is also given by several FMRI experiments showing that there is a distinct pattern of brain activity that occurs when people are experiencing different emotions. Zeki and Romaya, for example, investigated the neural correlates of hate with an FMRI procedure [108]. In their experiment, people had their brains scanned while viewing pictures of people they hated. The results showed increased activity in the medial frontal gyrus, right putamen, bilaterally in the premotor cortex, in the frontal pole, and bilaterally in the medial insula of the human brain. Also the activity of emotionally enhanced memory retention can be linked to human evolution [16]. During early development, in fact, responsive behavior to environmental events is likely to have progressed as a process of trial-and-error. Survival depended on behavioral patterns that were repeated or reinforced through life and death situations. Through evolution, this process of learning became genetically embedded in humans and all animal species in what is known as 'fight or flight' instinct [14].

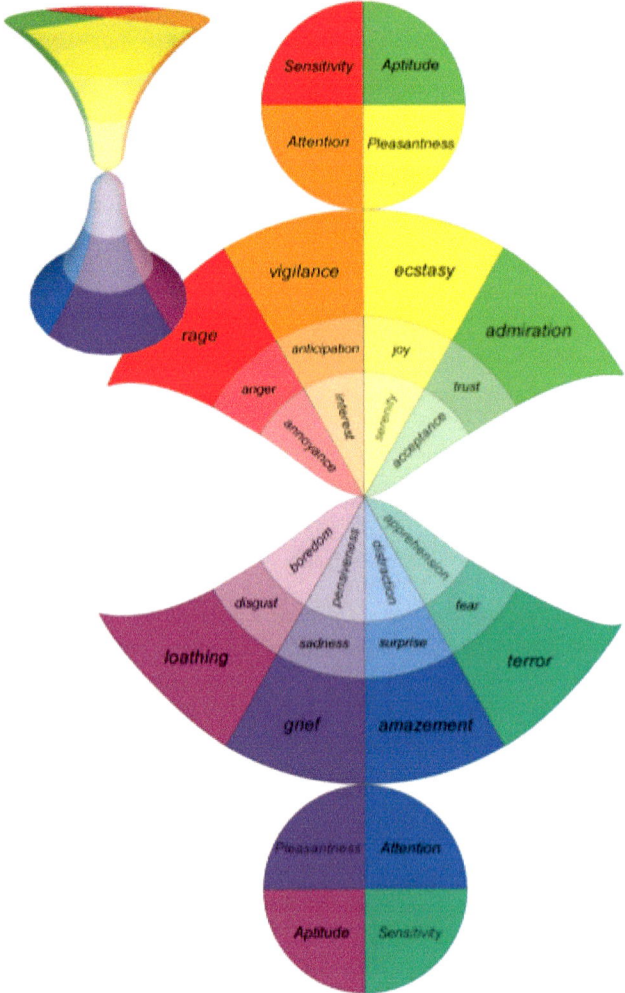

Fig. 3.17 The 3D model and the net of the Hourglass of Emotions. Since affective states go from strongly positive to null to strongly negative, the model assumes a hourglass shape (Source: [25])

The primary quantity we can measure about an emotion we feel is its strength. However, when we feel a strong emotion, it is because we feel a very specific emotion. And, conversely, we cannot feel a specific emotion like fear or amazement without that emotion being reasonably strong. For such reasons, the transition between different emotional states is modelled, within the same affective dimension, using the function $G(x) = 1 - \frac{1}{\sigma\sqrt{2\pi}}e^{-x^2/2\sigma^2}$ with $\sigma = 0.5$, for its symmetric inverted bell curve shape that quickly rises up towards the unit value (Fig. 3.18).

In particular, the function models how the level of activation of each affective dimension varies from the state of 'emotional void' (null value) to the state of

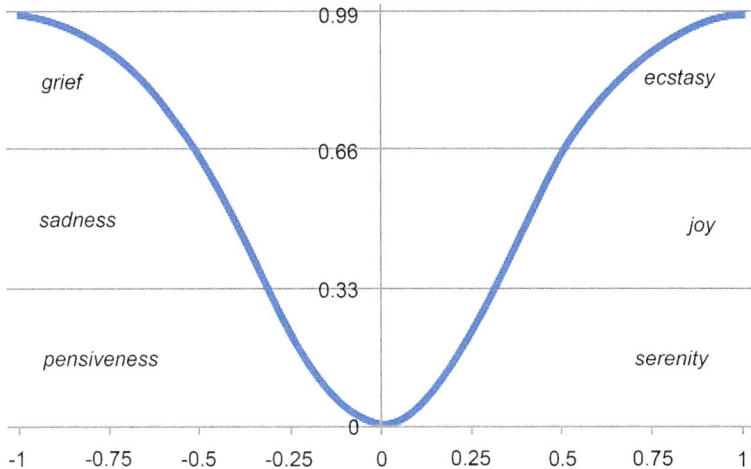

Fig. 3.18 The Pleasantness emotional flow. The passage from a sentic level to another is regulated by a Gaussian function that models how stronger emotions induce higher emotional sensitivity (Source: [25])

'heightened emotionality' (unit value). Justification for assuming that the Gaussian function (rather than a step or simple linear function) is appropriate for modeling the variation of emotion intensity is based on research into the neural and behavioral correlates of emotion, which are assumed to indicate emotional intensity in some sense. In fact, nobody genuinely knows what function subjective emotion intensity follows, because it has never been truly or directly measured [10]. For example, the so-called Duchenne smile (a genuine smile indicating pleasure) is characterized by smooth onset, increasing to an apex, and a smooth, relatively lengthy offset [58]. More generally, Klaus Scherer has argued that emotion is a process characterized by non-linear relations among its component elements – especially physiological measures, which typically look Gaussian [67]. Emotions, in fact, are not linear [88]: the stronger the emotion, the easier it is to be aware of it. Mapping this space of possible emotions leads to a hourglass shape.

It is worth to note that, in the model, the state of 'emotional void' is a-dimensional, which contributes to determine the hourglass shape. Total absence of emotion, in fact, can be associated with the total absence of reasoning (or, at least, consciousness) [35], which is not an envisaged mental state as, in the human mind, there is never nothing going on. The Hourglass of Emotions, in particular, can be exploited in the context of HCI to measure how much respectively: the user is amused by interaction modalities (Pleasantness), the user is interested in interaction contents (Attention), the user is comfortable with interaction dynamics (Sensitivity), the user is confident in interaction benefits (Aptitude). Each affective dimension, in particular, is characterized by six levels of activation (measuring the strength of an emotion), termed 'sentic levels', which represent the intensity thresholds of the expressed or perceived emotion. These levels are also labelled as a set of 24 basic

Table 3.7 The sentic levels of the Hourglass model. Labels are organized into four affective dimensions with six different levels each, whose combined activity constitutes the 'total state' of the mind (Source: [22])

Interval	Pleasantness	Attention	Sensitivity	Aptitude
[G(1), G(2/3))	Ecstasy	Vigilance	Rage	Admiration
[G(2/3), G(1/3))	Joy	Anticipation	Anger	Trust
[G(1/3), G(0))	Serenity	Interest	Annoyance	Acceptance
(G(0), G(−1/3)]	Pensiveness	Distraction	Apprehension	Boredom
(G(−1/3), G(−2/3)]	Sadness	Surprise	Fear	Disgust
(G(−2/3), G(−1)]	Grief	Amazement	Terror	Loathing

emotions [88], six for each of the affective dimensions, in a way that allows the model to specify the affective information associated with text both in a dimensional and in a discrete form (Table 3.7).

The dimensional form, in particular, is termed 'sentic vector' and it is a four-dimensional *float* vector that can potentially synthesize the full range of emotional experiences in terms of Pleasantness, Attention, Sensitivity, and Aptitude. In the model, the vertical dimension represents the intensity of the different affective dimensions, i.e., their level of activation, while the radial dimension represents K-lines [77] that can activate configurations of the mind, which can either last just a few seconds or years. The model follows the pattern used in color theory and research in order to obtain judgements about combinations, i.e., the emotions that result when two or more fundamental emotions are combined, in the same way that red and blue make purple.

Hence, some particular sets of sentic vectors have special names, as they specify well-known compound emotions (Fig. 3.19). For example, the set of sentic vectors with a level of Pleasantness $\in$ [G(2/3), G(1/3)), i.e., joy, a level of Aptitude $\in$ [G(2/3), G(1/3)), i.e., trust, and a minor magnitude of Attention and Sensitivity, are termed 'love sentic vectors' since they specify the compound emotion of love (Table 3.8). More complex emotions can be synthesized by using three, or even four, sentic levels, e.g., joy + trust + anger = jealousy.

Therefore, analogous to the way primary colors combine to generate different color gradations (and even colors we do not have a name for), the primary emotions of the Hourglass model can blend to form the full spectrum of human emotional experience. Beyond emotion detection, the Hourglass model is also used for polarity detection tasks. Since polarity is strongly connected to attitudes and feelings, in fact, it is defined in terms of the four affective dimensions, according to the formula:

$$p = \sum_{i=1}^{N} \frac{Pleasantness(c_i) + |Attention(c_i)| - |Sensitivity(c_i)| + Aptitude(c_i)}{9N}$$

(3.12)

where c_i is an input concept, N the total number of concepts, and 9 the normalization factor (as the Hourglass dimensions are defined as float $\in [-1,+1]$). In the formula,

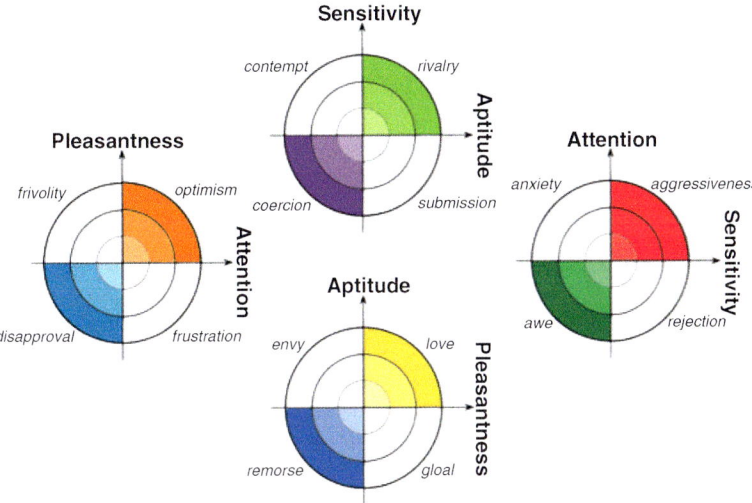

Fig. 3.19 Hourglass compound emotions of second level. By combining basic emotions pairwise, it is possible to obtain complex emotions resulting from the activation of two affective dimensions (Source: [25])

Table 3.8 The second-level emotions generated by pairwise combination of the sentic levels of the Hourglass model. The co-activation of different levels gives birth to different compound emotions (Source: [22])

	Attention>0	Attention<0	Aptitude>0	Aptitude<0
Pleasantness>0	Optimism	Frivolity	Love	Gloat
Pleasantness<0	Frustration	Disapproval	Envy	Remorse
Sensitivity>0	Aggressiveness	Rejection	Rivalry	Contempt
Sensitivity<0	Anxiety	Awe	Submission	Coercion

Attention is taken as absolute value since both its positive and negative intensity values correspond to positive polarity values (e.g., 'surprise' is negative in the sense of lack of Attention, but positive from a polarity point of view). Similarly, Sensitivity is taken as negative absolute value since both its positive and negative intensity values correspond to negative polarity values (e.g., 'anger' is positive in the sense of level of activation of Sensitivity, but negative in terms of polarity). The formula can be seen as one of the first attempts to show a clear connection between emotion recognition (sentiment analysis) and polarity detection (opinion mining).

3.3.3 Sentic Neurons

Affective analogical reasoning consists in processing the cognitive and affective information associated with natural language concepts, in order to compare the similarities between new and understood concepts and, hence, use such similarities to gain understanding of the new concept. It is a form of inductive reasoning because it strives to provide understanding of what is likely to be true, rather than deductively proving something as fact. The reasoning process begins by determining the target concept to be learned or explained. It is then compared to a general matching concept whose semantics and sentics (that is, the conceptual and affective information associated with it) are already well-understood. The two concepts must be similar enough to make a valid, substantial comparison.

Affective analogical reasoning is based on the brain's ability to form semantic patterns by association. The brain may be able to understand new concepts more easily if they are perceived as being part of a semantic pattern. If a new concept is compared to something the brain already knows, it may be more likely that the brain will store the new information more readily.

Such a semantic association needs *high generalization performance*, in order to better match conceptual and affective patterns. Because of the dynamic nature of AffectiveSpace, moreover, affective analogical reasoning should be characterized by *fast learning speed*, in order for concept associations to be recalculated every time a new multi-word expression is inserted in AffectNet. Finally, the process should be of *low computational complexity*, in order to perform big social data analysis [55]. All such features are those typical of extreme learning machine (ELM), a machine learning technique that, in recent years, has proved to be a powerful tool to tackle challenging modeling problems [21, 51].

3.3.3.1 Extreme Learning Machine

The ELM approach [53] was introduced to overcome some well-known issues in back-propagation network [91] training, specifically, potentially slow convergence rates, the critical tuning of optimization parameters [105], and the presence of local minima that call for multi-start and re-training strategies. The ELM learning problem settings require a training set, X, of N labeled pairs, where $(\mathbf{x}_i, y_i)$, where $\mathbf{x}_i \in \mathscr{R}^m$ is the i-th input vector and $y_i \in \mathscr{R}$ is the associate expected 'target' value; using a scalar output implies that the network has one output unit, without loss of generality.

The input layer has m neurons and connects to the 'hidden' layer (having N_h neurons) through a set of weights $\{\hat{\mathbf{w}}_j \in \mathscr{R}^m; j = 1, \ldots, N_h\}$. The j-th hidden neuron embeds a bias term, $\hat{b}_j$, and a nonlinear 'activation' function, $\varphi(\cdot)$; thus the neuron's response to an input stimulus, $\mathbf{x}$, is:

$$a_j(\mathbf{x}) = \varphi(\hat{\mathbf{w}}_j \cdot \mathbf{x} + \hat{b}_j) \qquad (3.13)$$

Note that (3.13) can be further generalized to a wider class of functions [52] but for the subsequent analysis this aspect is not relevant. A vector of weighted links, $\bar{\mathbf{w}}_j \in \mathscr{R}^{N_h}$, connects hidden neurons to the output neuron without any bias [50]. The overall output function, $f(\mathbf{x})$, of the network is:

$$f(\mathbf{x}) = \sum_{j=1}^{N_h} \bar{\mathbf{w}}_j a_j(\mathbf{x}) \tag{3.14}$$

It is convenient to define an 'activation matrix', $\mathbf{H}$, such that the entry $\{h_{ij} \in \mathbf{H}; i = 1, \ldots, N; j = 1, \ldots, N_h\}$ is the activation value of the j-th hidden neuron for the i-th input pattern. The $\mathbf{H}$ matrix is:

$$\mathbf{H} \equiv \begin{bmatrix} \varphi(\hat{\mathbf{w}}_1 \cdot \mathbf{x}_1 + \hat{b}_1) & \cdots & \varphi(\hat{\mathbf{w}}_{N_h} \cdot \mathbf{x}_1 + \hat{b}_{N_h}) \\ \vdots & \ddots & \vdots \\ \varphi(\hat{\mathbf{w}}_1 \cdot \mathbf{x}_N + \hat{b}_1) & \cdots & \varphi(\hat{\mathbf{w}}_{N_h} \cdot \mathbf{x}_N + \hat{b}_{N_h}) \end{bmatrix} \tag{3.15}$$

In the ELM model, the quantities $\{\hat{\mathbf{w}}_j, \hat{b}_j\}$ in (3.13) are set randomly and are not subject to any adjustment, and the quantities $\{\bar{\mathbf{w}}_j, \bar{b}\}$ in (3.14) are the only degrees of freedom. The training problem reduces to the minimization of the convex cost:

$$\min_{\{\bar{\mathbf{w}}, \bar{b}\}} \left\| \mathbf{H}\bar{\mathbf{w}} - \mathbf{y} \right\|^2 \tag{3.16}$$

A matrix pseudo-inversion yields the unique L_2 solution, as proven in [53]:

$$\bar{\mathbf{w}} = \mathbf{H}^+ \mathbf{y} \tag{3.17}$$

The simple, efficient procedure to train an ELM therefore involves the following steps:

1. Randomly set the input weights $\hat{\mathbf{w}}_i$ and bias $\hat{b}_i$ for each hidden neuron;
2. Compute the activation matrix, $\mathbf{H}$, as per (3.15);
3. Compute the output weights by solving a pseudo-inverse problem as per (3.17).

Despite the apparent simplicity of the ELM approach, the crucial result is that even random weights in the hidden layer endow a network with a notable representation ability [53]. Moreover, the theory derived in [54] proves that regularization strategies can further improve its generalization performance. As a result, the cost function (3.16) is augmented by an L_2 regularization factor as follows:

$$\min_{\bar{\mathbf{w}}} \{ \left\| \mathbf{H}\bar{\mathbf{w}} - \mathbf{y} \right\|^2 + \lambda \left\| \bar{\mathbf{w}} \right\|^2 \} \tag{3.18}$$

3.3.3.2 The Emotion Categorization Framework

The proposed framework [20] is designed to receive as input a natural language concept represented according to an M-dimensional space and to predict the corresponding sentic levels for the four affective dimensions involved: Pleasantness, Attention, Sensitivity, and Aptitude. The dimensionality M of the input space stems

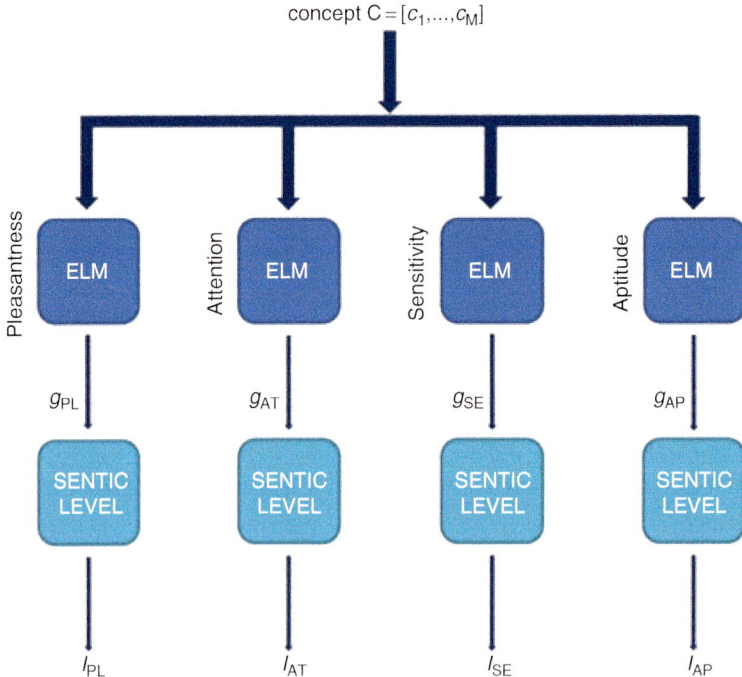

concept C = [c_1,...,c_M]

Pleasantness   ELM   Attention   ELM   Sensitivity   ELM   Aptitude   ELM

g_{PL} g_{AT} g_{SE} g_{AP}

SENTIC LEVEL   SENTIC LEVEL   SENTIC LEVEL   SENTIC LEVEL

l_{PL} l_{AT} l_{SE} l_{AP}

Fig. 3.20 The ELM-based framework for describing commonsense concepts in terms of the four Hourglass model's dimensions (Source: [89])

from the specific design of AffectiveSpace. As for the outputs, in principle each affective dimension can be characterized by an analog value in the range $[-1, 1]$, which represents the intensity of the expressed or received emotion.

Indeed, those analog values are eventually remapped to obtain six different sentic levels for each affective dimension. The categorization framework spans each affective dimension separately, under the reasonable assumption that the various dimensions map perceptual phenomena that are mutually independent [22]. As a result, each affective dimension is handled by a dedicated ELM, which addresses a regression problem.

Thus, each ELM-based predictor is fed by the M-dimensional vector describing the concept and yields as output the analog value that would eventually lead to the corresponding sentic level. Figure 3.20 provides the overall scheme of the framework; here, g_X is the level of activation predicted by the ELM and l_X is the corresponding sentic level. In theory, one might also implement the framework showed in Fig. 3.20 by using four independent predictors based on a multi-class classification schema. In such a case, each predictor would directly yield as output a sentic level out of the six available. However, two important aspects should be taken into consideration. First, the design of a reliable multi-class predictor is not straightforward, especially when considering that several alternative schemata have been proposed in the literature without a clearly established solution. Second, the emotion categorization scheme based on sentic levels stem from an inherently analog model, i.e., the Hourglass of Emotions. This ultimately motivates the choice of designing the four prediction systems as regression problems.

In fact, the framework schematized in Fig. 3.20 represents an intermediate step in the development of the final emotion categorization system. One should take into account that every affective dimension can in practice take on seven different values: the six available sentic levels plus a 'neutral' value, which in theory correspond to the value $G(0)$ in the Hourglass model. In practice, though, the neutral level is assigned to those concepts that are characterized by a level activation that lies in an interval around $G(0)$ in that affective dimension. Therefore, the final framework should properly manage the eventual seven-level scale. To this end, the complete categorization system is set to include a module that is able to predict if an affective dimension is present or absent in the description of a concept. In the latter case, no sentic level should be associated with that affective dimension (i.e., $I_x = $ null). This task is hereby addressed by exploiting the hierarchical approach presented in Fig. 3.21. Hence, given a concept and an affective dimension, first a SVM-based binary classifier is entitled to decide if a sentic level should be assessed. Accordingly, the ELM-based predictor is asked to assess the level of activation only if the SVM-based classifier determines that a sentic level should be associated with

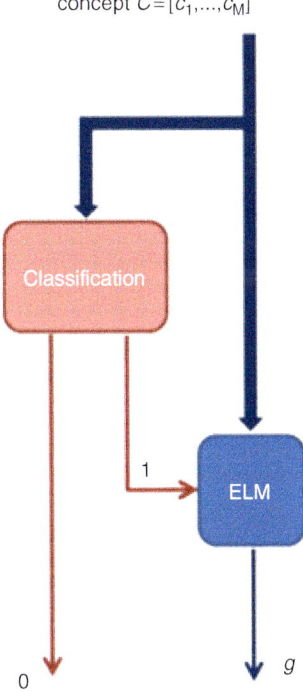

Fig. 3.21 The hierarchical scheme in which an SVM-based classifier first filters out unemotional concepts and an ELM-based predictor then classifies emotional concepts in terms of the involved affective dimension (Source: [89])

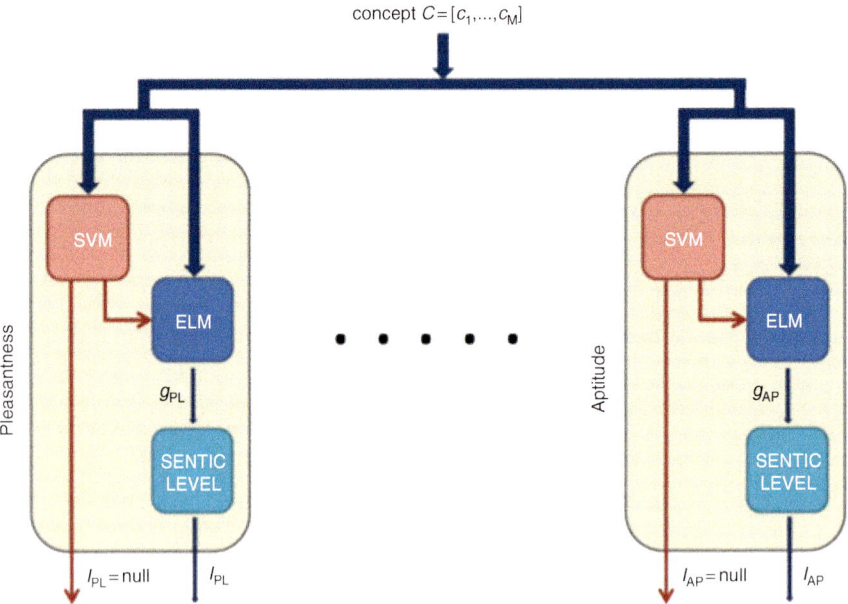

Fig. 3.22 The final framework: a hierarchical scheme is adopted to classify emotional concepts in terms of Pleasantness, Attention, Sensitivity, and Aptitude (Source: [89])

that concept. Otherwise, it is assumed that the neutral level should be associated with that concept (i.e., the corresponding affective dimension is not involved in the description of that concept). Obviously, such structure is replicated for each affective dimension. Figure 3.22 schematizes the complete framework.

3.3.3.3 Experimental Results

The proposed emotion categorization framework has been tested both on a benchmark of 6,813 commonsense concepts and on the real-world dataset of 2,000 patient opinions. As for the benchmark, the Sentic API was used to obtain for each concept the corresponding sentic vector, i.e., the level of activation of each affective dimension. According to the Hourglass model, the Sentic API expresses the level of activation as an analog number in the range $[-1, 1]$, which are eventually mapped into sentic levels by adopting the Gaussian mapping function. Indeed, the neutral sentic level is codified by the value '0'. The format adopted by the Sentic API to represent the levels of activation actually prevents one to approach the prediction problem as an authentic regression task, as per Fig. 3.20.

The neutral sentic level corresponds to a single value in the analog range used to represent activations. Therefore, experimental results are presented as follows: firstly, the performance of the system depicted in Fig. 3.20 is analyzed (according to that set-up, the ELM-based predictors are not designed to assess the neutral sentic level); secondly, the performance of the complete framework (Fig. 3.22) is discussed; lastly, a use-case evaluation on the patient opinion dataset is proposed.

3.3.3.4 Accuracy in the Prediction of the Sentic Levels

The emotion categorization framework proposed in Fig. 3.20 exploits four independent ELM-based predictors to estimate the levels of activation of as many affective dimensions. In this experiment, it is assumed that each ELM-based predictor can always assess correctly a level of activation set to '0'. A cross-validation procedure has been used to robustly evaluate the performance of the framework.

As a result, the experimental session involved ten different experimental runs. In each run, 800 concepts randomly extracted from the complete benchmark provided the test set; the remaining concepts were heavenly split into a training set and a validation set. The validation set was designed to support the model selection phase, i.e., the selection of the best parameterization for the ELM predictors. In the present configuration, two quantities were involved in the model selection phase: the number of neurons N_h in the hidden layer and the regularization parameter λ.

The following parameters were used for model selection:

- $N_h \in [100, 1,000]$ by steps of 100 neurons;
- $\lambda = \{1 \cdot 10^{-6}, 1 \cdot 10^{-5}, 1 \cdot 10^{-4}, 1 \cdot 10^{-3}, 1 \cdot 10^{-2}, 1 \cdot 10^{-1}, 1\}$.

In each run the performance of the emotion categorization framework was measured by using only the patterns included in the test set, i.e., the patterns that were not involved in the training phase or in the model selection phase. Table 3.9 reports the performance obtained by the emotion categorization framework over the ten runs. The table actually compares the results of three different sets up, which differs in the dimensionality M of AffectiveSpace that describe the concepts. Thus, Table 3.9 provides the results achieved with $M = 100$, $M = 70$, and $M = 50$.

The results refer to a configuration of the ELM predictors characterized by the following parameterization: $N_h = 200$ and $\lambda = 1$; such configuration was obtained by exploiting the model selection phase. The performance of each setting is evaluated according to the following quantities (expressed as average values over the ten runs):

- *Pearson's correlation coefficient*: the measure of the linear correlation between predicted levels of activation and expected levels of activation for the four predictors.
- *Strict accuracy*: the percentage of patterns for which the framework correctly predicted the four sentic levels; thus, a concept is assumed to be correctly classified only if the predicted sentic level corresponds to the expected sentic level for every affective dimension.
- *Smooth accuracy*: the percentage of patterns for which the framework correctly predicted three sentic levels out of four; thus, a concept is assumed to be correctly classified even when one among the four predictors fails to assign the correct sentic level.

Table 3.9 Performance obtained by the emotion categorization framework over the ten runs with three different set-ups of AffectiveSpace (Source: [22])

M	Correlation				Accuracy		
	Pleasantness	Attention	Sensitivity	Aptitude	Strict	Smooth	Relaxed
100	0.69	0.67	0.78	0.72	39.4	73.4	87.0
70	0.71	0.67	0.78	0.72	41.0	75.4	88.4
50	0.66	0.66	0.77	0.71	40.9	75.3	86.4

- *Relaxed accuracy*: in this case, one relaxes the definition of correct prediction of the sentic level. As a result, given an affective dimension, the prediction is assumed correct even when the assessed sentic level and the expected sentic level are contiguous in Table 3.7. As an example, let suppose that the expected sentic level in the affective dimension Sensitivity for the incoming concept is 'annoyance'. Then, the prediction is assumed correct even when the assessed sentic level is 'anger' or 'apprehension'. Therefore, the relaxed accuracy gives the percentage of patterns for which the framework correctly predicted the four sentic levels according to such criterion.

In practice, the smooth accuracy and the relaxed accuracy allow one to take into account two crucial issues: the dataset can include noise and entries may incorporate a certain degree of subjectiveness. The results provided in Table 3.9 lead to the following comments:

- Emotion categorization is in fact a challenging problem; in this regard, the gap between strict accuracy and smooth/relaxed accuracies confirms that the presence of noise is a crucial issue.
- The ELM-based framework can attain satisfactory performance in terms of smooth accuracy and relaxed accuracy. Actually, the proposed framework scored a 75% accuracy in correctly assessing at least three affective dimension for an input concept.
- Reliable performance can be achieved even when a 50-dimensional AffectiveSpace is used to characterize concepts. The latter result indeed represents a very interesting outcome, as previous approaches to the same problem in general exploited a 100-dimensional AffectiveSpace. In this respect, the present work shows that the use of ELM-based predictors can reduce the overall complexity of the framework by shrinking the feature space.

3.3.3.5 Accuracy of the Complete Emotion Categorization System

The complete categorization system exploits the hierarchical approach presented in Fig. 3.21 to assess the level of activation of a concept. According to such a set-up, the accuracy of the SVM-based classifier is critical to the whole system's performance, as it handles the preliminary filtering task before that actual sentic description is evaluated. In principle, one might analyze the performance of the two components separately and assess the run-time generalization accuracy accordingly. Nevertheless, in the present context, the system performance has been measured as a whole, irrespectively of the internal structure of the evaluation scheme. On the other hand, one should also consider that, given a concept and a sentic dimension in which such concept should be assessed as neutral, to predict a low activation value is definitely less critical than predicting a large activation value.

Therefore, the system performance has been evaluated by avoiding considering as an error the cases in which the expected sentic level is 'neutral' and the assessed sentic level is the less intense (either positive or negative). As an example, given the sentic dimension Attention, to classify a neutral sentic level either as 'interest' or 'distraction' would not be considered an error. The performance of the framework has been evaluated by exploiting the same cross-validation approach already applied in the previous experimental session. In the present case, though, the model selection approach involved both the SVM-based classifiers and the ELM-based predictors. For the SVM classifiers, two quantities were set with model selection: the regularization parameter C and the width σ of the Gaussian kernel. The following parameters were used for model selection:

- $C = \{1, 10, 100, 1,000\}$;
- $\sigma = \{0.1, 0.25, 0.5, 0.75, 1, 1.5, 2, 5, 10\}$.

The performance obtained by the framework over the ten runs was of 38.3%, 72%, and 79.8%, for strict accuracy, smooth accuracy, and relaxed accuracy, respectively. In this case, the experimental session involved only the set-up $M = 50$, which already proved to attain a satisfactory trade-off between accuracy and complexity.

The results refer to a configuration of the SVM classifiers characterized by the following parameterization: $C = 1$ and $\sigma = 1.5$. As expected, the accuracy of the complete framework is slightly inferior to that of the system presented in the previous section. Indeed, the results confirm that the proposed approach can attain satisfactory accuracies by exploiting a 50-dimensional AffectiveSpace. In this regard, one should also notice that the estimated performance of the proposed methodology appears quite robust, as it is estimated on ten independent runs involving different compositions of the training and the test set.

3.4   Semantic Parsing

3.4.1   *Pre-processing*

Before text can be parsed, it needs to be normalized. To this end, a pre-processing module interprets all the affective valence indicators usually contained in opinionated text such as special punctuation, complete upper-case words, onomatopoeic repetitions, exclamation words, degree adverbs and emoticons. At the moment, this is done mainly by replacing fixed social expressions with their normalized version stored in a database of common patterns.

3.4.2   *Concept Extraction*

Concept extraction [90] is about breaking text into clauses and, hence, deconstruct such clauses into bags of concepts, in order to feed these into a commonsense reasoning algorithm. For applications in fields such as real-time HCI and big social data analysis, in fact, deep natural language understanding is not strictly required: a sense of the semantics associated with text and some extra information (affect) associated with such semantics are often enough to quickly perform tasks such as emotion recognition and polarity detection.

3.4.2.1   From Sentence to Verb and Noun Chunks

The first step in the proposed algorithm breaks text into clauses. Each verb and its associated noun phrase are considered in turn, and one or more concepts is extracted from these. As an example, the clause "I went for a walk in the park", would contain the concepts *go walk* and *go park*. The Stanford Chunker [73] is used to chunk the input text. A sentence like "I am going to the market to buy vegetables and some fruits" would be broken into "I am going to the market" and "to buy vegetables and some fruits". A general assumption during clause separation is that, if a piece of text contains a preposition or subordinating conjunction, the words preceding these function words are interpreted not as events but as objects. The next step of the algorithm then separates clauses into verb and noun chunks, as suggested by the following parse tree:

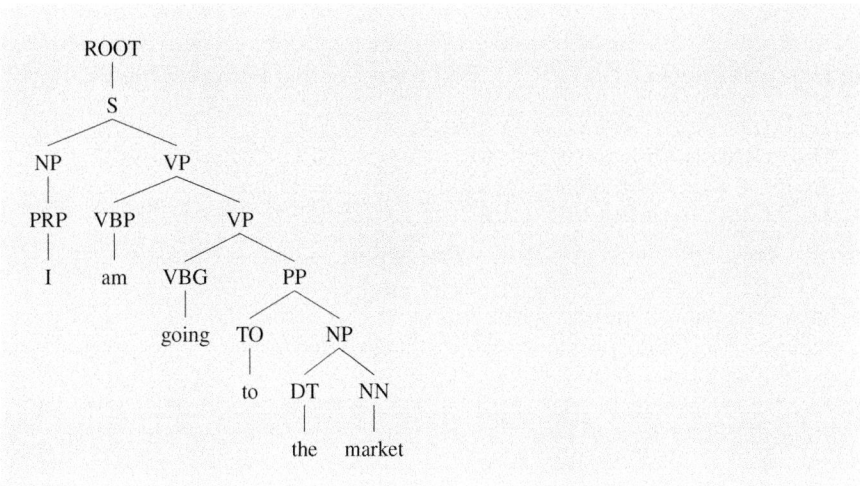

and

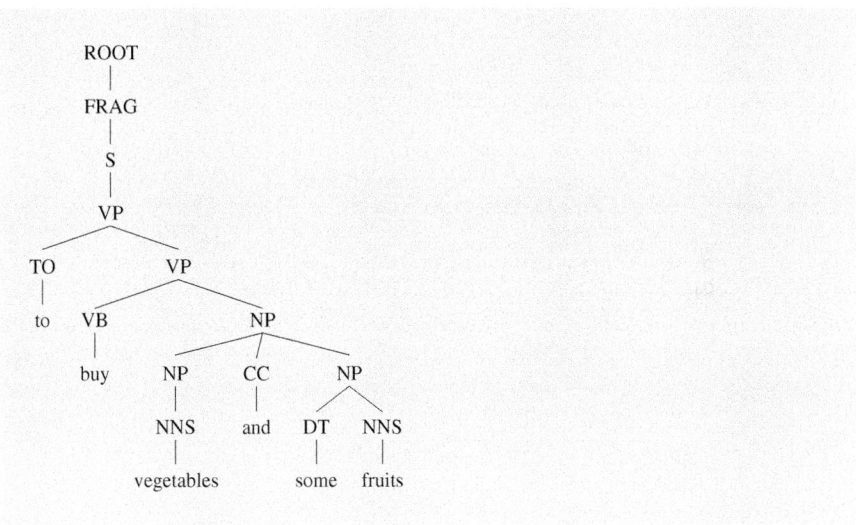

3.4.2.2 Obtaining the Full List of Concepts

Next, clauses are normalized in two stages. First, each *verb* chunk is normalized using the Stanford lemmatization algorithm. Second, each potential *noun* chunk associated with individual verb chunks is paired with the lemmatized verb in order to detect multi-word expressions of the form 'verb plus object'. Objects alone, however, can also represent a commonsense concept. To detect such expressions, a

POS-based bigram algorithm checks noun phrases for stopwords and adjectives. In particular, noun phrases are first split into bigrams and then processed through POS patterns, as shown in Algorithm 3.1. POS pairs are taken into account as follows:

1. ADJECTIVE NOUN: The adj+noun combination and noun as a stand-alone concept are added to the objects list.
2. ADJECTIVE STOPWORD: The entire bigram is discarded.
3. NOUN ADJECTIVE: As trailing adjectives do not tend to carry sufficient information, the adjective is discarded and only the noun is added as a valid concept.
4. NOUN NOUN: When two nouns occur in sequence, they are considered to be part of a single concept. Examples include *butter scotch*, *ice cream*, *cream biscuit*, and so on.
5. NOUN STOPWORD : The stopword is discarded, and only the noun is considered valid.
6. STOPWORD ADJECTIVE: The entire bigram is discarded.

Algorithm 3.1: POS-based bigram algorithm

Data: NounPhrase
  Result: Valid object concepts
  Split the NounPhrase into bigrams ;
  Initialize concepts to Null ;
  for *each NounPhrase* **do**
      while *For every* bigram *in the NounPhrase* **do**
          POS Tag the Bigram ;
          if adj noun **then**
          | add to Concepts: noun, adj+noun

          else if noun noun **then**
          | add to Concepts: noun+noun

          else if stopword noun **then**
          | add to Concepts: noun

          else if adj stopword **then**
          | continue

          else if stopword adj **then**
          | continue

          else
          | Add to Concepts : entire bigram
          end
          repeat until no more bigrams left;
      end
  end

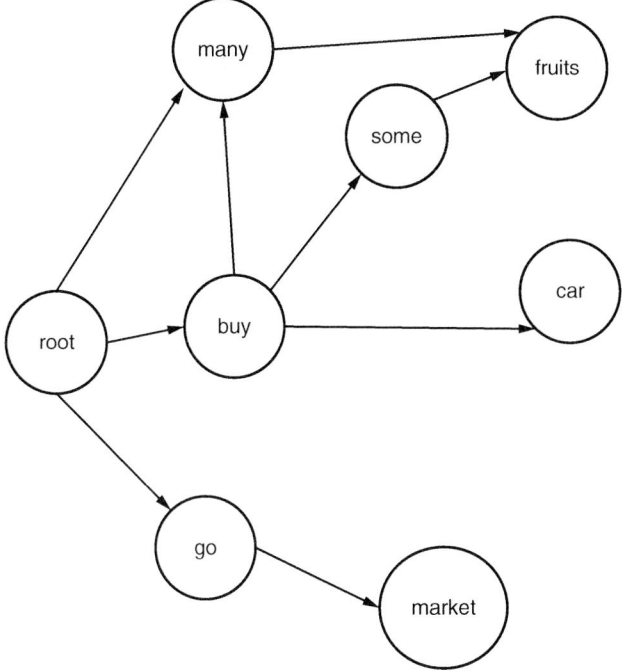

Fig. 3.23 Example parse graph for multi-word expressions (Source: [90])

7. STOPWORD NOUN: In bigrams matching this pattern, the stopword is discarded and the noun alone qualifies as a valid concept.

The POS-based bigram algorithm extracts concepts such as *market, some fruits, fruits,* and *vegetables.* In order to capture event concepts, matches between the object concepts and the normalized verb chunks are searched. This is done by exploiting a parse graph that maps all the multi-word expressions contained in the knowledge bases (Fig. 3.23). Such an unweighted directed graph helps to quickly detect multi-word concepts, without performing an exhaustive search throughout all the possible word combinations that can form a commonsense concept. Single-word concepts, e.g., *house,* that already appear in the clause as a multi-word concept, e.g., *beautiful house,* in fact, are pleonastic (providing redundant information) and are discarded. In this way, the Algorithm 3.2 is able to extract event concepts such as *go market, buy some fruits, buy fruits,* and *buy vegetables,* representing bags of concepts to be fed to a commonsense reasoning algorithm for further processing.

Algorithm 3.2: Event concept extraction algorithm

Data: Natural language sentence
  Result: List of concepts
  Find the number of verbs in the sentence;
  for *every clause* **do**
      extract VerbPhrases and NounPhrases;
      lemmatize VERB ;
      for *every NounPhrase with the associated verb* **do**
          find possible forms of *objects* ;
          link all *objects* to lemmatized verb to get *events*;
      end
      repeat until no more clauses are left;
  end

3.4.3   Similarity Detection

Because natural language concepts may be expressed in a multitude of forms, it is necessary to have a technique for defining the similarity of multi-word expressions so that a concept can be detected in all its different forms. The main aim of the proposed similarity detection technique, in fact, is to find concepts that are both syntactically and semantically related to the ones generated by the event concept extraction algorithm, in order to make up for concepts for which no matches are found in the knowledge bases. In particular, the POS tagging based bigram algorithm is employed to calculate syntactic matches, while the knowledge bases are exploited to find semantic matches. Beyond this, concept similarity may be exploited to merge concepts in the database and thus reduce data sparsity. When commonsense data is collected from different data sources, in fact, the same concepts tend to appear in different forms and merging these can be key for enhancing the commonsense reasoning capabilities of the system.

3.4.3.1   Syntactic Match Step

The syntactic match step checks whether two concepts have at least one object in common. For each noun phrase, objects and their matches from the knowledge bases are extracted, providing a collection of related properties for specific concepts. All the matching properties for each noun phrase are collected separately. The sets are then compared in order to identify common elements. If common elements exist, phrases are considered to be similar. Such similarity is deduced as shown in Algorithm 3.3.

Algorithm 3.3: Finding similar concepts

Data: NounPhrase1, NounPhrase2
  Result: *True* if the concepts are similar, else *False*
  if *Both phrases have atleast one* noun *in common* **then**
      Objects1 := All Valid Objects for NounPhrase1;
      Objects2 := All Valid Objects for NounPhrase2;
      M1 = matches from KB for
      M1 := ∅ ;
      M2 := ∅ ;
      for *all* concepts *in NounPhrase1* **do**
          M1 := M1 ∪ *all property matches for concept*;
      end
      for *all* concepts *in NounPhrase2* **do**
          M2 := M2 ∪ *all property matches for concept* ;
      end
      SetCommon = M1 ∪ M2 ;
      if *length of* SetCommon > *0* **then**
          The Noun Phrases are similar
      else
          They are not similar
      end

3.4.3.2 Semantic Similarity Detection

Semantic similarity is calculated by means of AffectiveSpace and sentic medoids. In particular, in order to measure such semantic relatedness, AffectiveSpace is clustered by using a k-medoid approach [87]. Unlike the k-means algorithm (which does not pose constraints on centroids), k-medoids do assume that centroids must coincide with k observed points. The k-medoids approach is similar to the partitioning around medoids (PAM) algorithm, which determines a medoid for each cluster selecting the most centrally located centroid within that cluster. Unlike other PAM techniques, however, the k-medoids algorithm runs similarly to k-means and, hence, requires a significantly reduced computational time. Given that the distance between two points in the space is defined as $D(e_i, e_j) = \sqrt{\sum_{s=1}^{d'} \left(e_i^{(s)} - e_j^{(s)} \right)^2}$, the adopted algorithm can be summarized as follows:

1. Each centroid $\bar{e}_i \in \mathbb{R}^{d'}$ ($i = 1, 2, \ldots, k$) is set as one of the k most representative instances of general categories such as time, location, object, animal, and plant;
2. Assign each instance e_j to a cluster $\bar{e}_i$ if $D(e_j, \bar{e}_i) \leq D(e_j, \bar{e}_{i'})$ where $i(i') = 1, 2, \ldots, k$;

3. Find a new centroid $\bar{e}_i$ for each cluster c so that $\sum_{j \in Cluster\, c} D(e_j, \bar{e}_i) \leq \sum_{j \in Cluster\, c} D(e_j, \bar{e}_{i'})$;
4. Repeat step 2 and 3 until no changes are observed.

3.5 ELM Classifier

Despite being much more efficient than BoW and BoC models, sentic patterns are still limited by the richness of the knowledge base and the set of dependency-based rules. The main problem with ELM is in training them to work in the event of a large number of available samples, where the generalization performance has to be carefully assessed. For this reason, [83] proposes an ELM implementation that exploits the Spark distributed in memory technology and show how to take advantage of the most recent advances in SLT in order to address the issue of selecting ELM hyperparameters that give the best generalization performance. To be able to make a good guess even when no sentic pattern is matched or SenticNet entry found, the system resorts to machine learning. In particular, three well-known sentiment analysis datasets (Sect. 3.5.1), a set of four features per sentence (Sect. 3.5.2), and an artificial neural network (ANN) classifier (Sect. 3.5.3) are used to label text segments as positive or negative.

3.5.1 Datasets Used

3.5.1.1 Movie Review Dataset

The first dataset is derived from the benchmark corpus developed by Pang and Lee [85]. This corpus includes 1,000 positive and 1,000 negative movie reviews authored by expert movie reviewers, collected from rottentomatos.com, with all text converted to lowercase and lemmatized, and HTML tags removed. Originally, Pang and Lee manually labeled each review as positive or negative. Later, Socher et al. [96] annotated this dataset at sentence level. They extracted 11,855 sentences from the reviews and manually labeled them using a fine grained inventory of five sentiment labels: *strong positive*, *positive*, *neutral*, *negative*, and *strong negative*. Since, this experiment is only about binary classification, sentences marked as neutral we removed and reduced the labels on the remaining sentences to positive or negative. Thus, the final movie dataset contained 9,613 sentences, of which 4,800 were labeled as positive and 4,813 as negative.

3.5.1.2   Blitzer Dataset

The second dataset is derived from the resource put together by Blitzer et al. [13], which consists of product reviews in seven different domains. For each domain there are 1,000 positive and 1,000 negative reviews. Only the reviews under the *electronics* category were used. From these 7,210 non-neutral sentences, 3,505 sentences from positive reviews and 3,505 from negative ones were randomly extracted, and manually annotated as positive or negative. Note that the polarity of individual sentences does not always coincide with the overall polarity of the review: for example, some negative reviews contain sentences such as "This is a good product – sounds great", "Gets good battery life", "Everything you'd hope for in an iPod dock" or "It is very cheap".

3.5.1.3   Amazon Product Review Dataset

The reviews of 453 mobile phones from http://amazon.com were crawled. Each review was split into sentences, and each sentence then manually labelled by its sentiment labels. Finally, 115,758 sentences were obtained, out of which 48,680 were negative, 2,957 sentences neutral and 64,121 positive. In this experiment, only positive and negative sentences employed. Hence, the final *Amazon dataset* contained 112,801 sentences annotated as either positive or negative.

3.5.2   Feature Set

3.5.2.1   Commonsense Knowledge Features

Commonsense knowledge features consist of concepts represented by means of AffectiveSpace. In particular, concepts extracted from text through the semantic parser are encoded as 100-dimensional real-valued vectors and then aggregated into a single vector representing the sentence by coordinate-wise summation: $x_i = \sum_{j=1}^{N} x_{ij}$, where x_i is the i-th coordinate of the sentence's feature vector, $i = 1, \ldots, 100$; x_{ij} is the i-th coordinate of its j-th concept's vector, and N is the number of concepts in the sentence.

3.5.2.2   Sentic Feature

The polarity scores of each concept extracted from the sentence were obtained from SenticNet and summed up to produce a single scalar feature.

3.5.2.3   Part-of-Speech Feature

The number of adjectives, adverbs, and nouns in the sentence; three separate features.

3.5.2.4   Modification Feature

This is a single binary feature. For each sentence, its dependency tree was obtained from the dependency parser. This tree was analyzed to determine whether there is any word modified by a noun, adjective, or adverb. The modification feature is set to 1 in case of any modification relation in the sentence; 0 otherwise.

3.5.2.5   Negation Feature

Similarly, the negation feature is a single binary feature determined by the presence of any negation in the sentence. It is important because the negation can invert the polarity of the sentence.

3.5.3   Classification

Sixty percent of the sentences were selected from each of the three datasets as the training set for the classification. The sentences from each dataset were randomly drawn in such a way to balance the dataset with 50% negative sentences and 50% positive sentences. Again, ELM was used, which was found to outperform a state-of-the-art SVM in terms of both accuracy and training time. An overall 71.32% accuracy was obtained on the Final Dataset described in Table 3.10 using ELM and 68.35% accuracy using SVM. The classifiers were also trained on each single dataset and tested over all the other datasets. Table 3.11 reports the comparative performance results obtained in this experiment. It can be noted from Table 3.11 that the model trained on the Amazon dataset produced the best accuracy compared to the movie review and Blitzer-derived datasets. For each of these experiments, ELM outperformed SVM. The best performance by the ELM classifier was obtained on the movie review dataset, while the SVM classifier performed best on the Blitzer dataset. The training and test set collected from different datasets are shown in Table 3.10. Hence, whenever a sentence cannot be processed by SenticNet and sentic patterns, the ELM classifier makes a good guess about sentence polarity, based on the available features. Although the ELM classifier has performed best when all features were used together, commonsense-knowledge based features resulted in the most significant ones. From the Table 3.12, it can be noticed that negation is also a useful feature. The other features were not found to have a significant role in the performance of the classifier but were still found to be useful for producing optimal

Table 3.10 Dataset to train and test ELM classifiers (Source: [89])

Dataset	Number of training sentences	Number of test sentences
Movie review dataset	5,678	3,935
Blitzer-derived dataset	4,326	2,884
Amazon dataset	67,681	45,120
Final dataset	77,685	51,939

Table 3.11 Performance of the classifiers: SVM/ELM classifier (Source: [89])

Training dataset	On movie review dataset	On Blitzer dataset	On Amazon dataset
Movie review	–	64.12%/72.12%	65.14%/69.21%
Blitzer	61.25%/68.09%	–	62.25%/66.73%
Amazon	69.77%/70.03%	72.23%/73.30%	–

Table 3.12 Feature analysis (Source: [89])

Features used	Accuracy (%)	Features used	Accuracy (%)
All	71.32	All except part-of-speech feature	70.41
All except commonsense	40.11	All except modification feature	71.53
All except sentic feature	70.84	All except negation feature	68.97

accuracy. As ELM provided the best accuracy, Table 3.12 presents the accuracy of the ELM classifier. It should be noted that since the main purpose of this work is to demonstrate the ensemble use of linguistic rules, a detailed investigative study on features and their relative impact on ELM classifiers is proposed for future work, to further enrich and optimize the performance of the ensemble framework.

3.5.4 Discussion

The discussed framework outperforms the state-of-the-art methods on both the movie review and the Amazon datasets and shows even better results on the Blitzer-derived dataset. This shows that the framework is robust and not biased towards a particular domain. Moreover, while standard statistical methods require extensive training, both in terms of resources (training corpora) and time (learning time), sentic patterns are mostly unsupervised, except for the ELM module, which is, though, very fast, due to the use of ELM. The addition and improvement of the patterns, as noted in [89], has helped the system improve its results. Results show performance improvement over [89]. On the other hand, [96] has failed to obtain consistently good accuracy over both Blitzer and amazon datasets but obtained good accuracy over the movie review dataset. This is because the classifier proposed in [96] was trained on the movie review dataset only. The proposed approach has therefore obtained a better accuracy than the baseline system. The three datasets described in Sects. 3.5.1.1, 3.5.1.2 and 3.5.1.3 were combined to evaluate the sentic

Table 3.13 Performance of the proposed system on sentences with conjunctions and comparison with state-of-the-art (Source: [89])

System	AND (%)	BUT (%)
Socher et al. [96]	84.26	39.79
Poria et al. [89]	87.91	84.17
Extended sentic patterns	**88.24**	**85.63**

patterns. From Sect. 3.5.1, the number of positive and negative sentences in the dataset can be calculated: this shows 72,721 positive and 56,903 negative sentences. If the system predicts all sentences as positive, this would give a baseline accuracy of 56.10%. Clearly, the proposed system performed well above than the baseline system. It is worth noting that the accuracy of the system crucially depends on the quality of the output of the dependency parser, which relies on grammatical correctness of the input sentences. All datasets, however, contain ungrammatical sentences which penalize results. On the other hand, the formation of a balanced dataset for ELM classifiers actually has a strong impact on developing a more accurate classifier than the one reported in Poria et al. [89].

3.5.4.1 Effect of Conjunctions

Sentiment is often very hard to identify when sentences have conjunctions. The performance of the proposed system was tested on two types of conjunctions: *and* and *but*. High accuracy was achieved for both conjunctions. However, the accuracy on sentences containing *but* was somewhat lower as some sentences of this type do not match sentic patterns. Just over 27% of the sentences in the dataset have *but* as a conjunction, which implies that the rule for *but* has a very significant impact on the accuracy. Table 3.13 shows the accuracy of the proposed system on sentences with *but* and *and* compared with the state of the art. The accuracy is averaged over all datasets.

3.5.4.2 Effect of Discourse Markers

Lin et al.'s [69] discourse parser was used to analyze the discourse structure of sentences. Out of the 1,211 sentences in the movie review and the Blitzer dataset that contain discourse markers (*though, although, despite*), sentiment was correctly identified in 85.67% sentences. According to Poria et al. [89], the discourse parser sometimes failed to detect the discourse structure of sentences such as *So, although the movie bagged a lot, I give very low rating.* Such problems were overcome by removing the occurrence of any word before the discourse marker when a discourse marker occurs at either second or third position in the sentence.

3.5.4.3 Effect of Negation

With the linguistic rules, negation was detected and its impact on sentence polarity was studied. Overall, 93.84% accuracy was achieved on polarity detection from sentences with negation. Socher et al. [96] state that negation does not always reverse the polarity. According to them, the sentence "I do not like the movie" does not bear any negative sentiment, being neutral. For "The movie is not terrible," their theory suggests that this sentence does not say that the movie is good but rather says that it is less bad, so this sentence bears negative sentiment. In the proposed annotation, this theory was not followed. The expression "not bad" was consider as implying satisfaction; thus, such a sentence was annotated as positive. Conversely, "not good" implies dissatisfaction and thus bears negative sentiment. Following this, the sentence "The movie is not terrible" is considered to be positive.

3.5.4.4 Examples of Differences Between the Proposed System and State-of-the-Art Approaches

Table 3.14 shows examples of various linguistic patterns and the performance of the proposed system across different sentence structures. Examples in Table 3.15 show that the proposed system produces consistent results on sentences carrying the same meaning although they use different words. In this example, the negative sentiment bearing word in the sentence is changed: in the first variant it is **bad**, in the second variant it is **bored**, and in the third variant it is **upset**. In each case, the system detects the sentiment correctly. This analysis also illustrates inconsistency of state-of-the-art approaches, given that the system [96] achieves the highest accuracy compared with other existing state-of-the-art systems.

Table 3.14 Performance comparison of the proposed system and state-of-the art approaches on different sentence structures (Source: [89])

Sentence	Socher et al. [96]	Sentic patterns
Hate iphone with a passion	Positive	Negative
Drawing has never been such easy in computer	Negative	Positive
The room is so small to stay	Neutral	Negative
The tooth hit the pavement and broke	Positive	Negative
I am one of the least happy people in the world	Neutral	Negative
I love starbucks but they just lost a customer	Neutral	Negative
I doubt that he is good	Positive	Negative
Finally, for the beginner there are not enough conceptual clues on what is actually going on	Positive	Negative
I love to see that he got injured badly	Neutral	Positive
I love this movie though others say it's bad	Neutral	Positive
Nothing can be better than this	Negative	Positive
The phone is very big to hold	Neutral	Negative

Table 3.15 Performance of the system on sentences bearing same meaning with different words (Source: [89])

Sentence	Socher et al. [96]	Sentic patterns
I feel **bad** when Messi scores fantastic goals	Neutral	Negative
I feel **bored** when Messi scores fantastic goals	Negative	Negative
I feel **upset** when Messi scores fantastic goals	Positive	Negative
I gave her a **gift**	Neutral	Positive
I gave her **poison**	Neutral	Negative

Table 3.16 Results obtained using SentiWordNet (Source: [89])

Dataset	Using SenticNet (%)	Using SentiWordNet (%)
Movie review	88.12	87.63
Blitzer	88.27	88.09
Amazon	82.75	80.28

3.5.4.5 Results Obtained Using SentiWordNet

An extensive experiment using SentiWordNet instead of SenticNet was carried out on all the three datasets. The results showed SenticNet performed slightly better than SentiWordNet. A possible future direction of this work is the invention of a novel approach to combine SenticNet and SentiWordNet in the sentiment analysis framework. The slight difference in the accuracy reported in Table 3.16 confirmed that both the lexicons share similar knowledge but since SenticNet contains concepts, this helps increase accuracy. For example, in the sentence "The battery lasts little", the proposed algorithm extracts the concept "last little" which exists in SenticNet but not in SentiWordNet. As a result, when SenticNet is used the framework labels the sentence with a "negative" sentiment but when using SentiWordNet the sentence is labeled with a "neutral" sentiment.

The next Chap. 3 introduces to how SenticNet as a resource is built. In particular, the chapter thoroughly explains the processes of knowledge acquisition, representation, and reasoning, which contribute to the generation of the semantics and sentics that form SenticNet

3.5.4.6 Examples of Cases When ELM Was Used

Table 3.17 presents some examples where ELM was used to guess the polarity. For each of these sentences, no concept was found in SenticNet.

Table 3.17 Some examples where ELM was used to obtain the polarity label (Source: [89])

Sentence	Polarity
I had to return the phone after 2 days of use	Negative
The phone runs recent operating system	Positive
The phone has a big and capacitive touchscreen	Positive
My iphone battery lasts only few hours	Negative
I remember that I slept at the movie hall	Negative

The next Chap. 4 introduces to the application of bio-medical domain lexicons. It describes how WME is built as a resource and the applications of WME as a standalone sentiment lexicon. This chapter dives into computation creativity and its application in machine learning to find the best K in K-Means.

References

1. Achlioptas, D.: Database-friendly random projections: Johnson-lindenstrauss with binary coins. J. Comput. Syst. Sci. **66**(4), 671–687 (2003)
2. Addis, M., Boch, L., Allasia, W., Gallo, F., Bailer, W., Wright, R.: 100 million hours of audiovisual content: digital preservation and access in the PrestoPRIME project. In: Digital Preservation Interoperability Framework Symposium, Dresden (2010)
3. von Ahn, L.: Games with a purpose. IEEE Comput. Mag. **6**, 92–94 (2006)
4. von Ahn, L., Dabbish, L.: Labeling images with a computer game. In: CHI, Vienna, pp. 319–326 (2004)
5. von Ahn, L., Ginosar, S., Kedia, M., Liu, R., Blum, M.: Improving accessibility of the web with a computer game. In: CHI, Quebec, pp. 79–82 (2006)
6. von Ahn, L., Kedia, M., Blum, M.: Verbosity: a game for collecting commonsense facts. In: CHI, Quebec, pp. 75–78 (2006)
7. von Ahn, L., Liu, R., Blum, M.: Peekaboom: a game for locating objects in images. In: CHI, pp. 55–64 (2006)
8. Ailon, N., Chazelle, B.: Faster dimension reduction. Commun. ACM **53**(2), 97–104 (2010)
9. Balduzzi, D.: Randomized co-training: from cortical neurons to machine learning and back again. (2013). arXiv preprint arXiv:1310.6536
10. Barrett, L.: Solving the emotion paradox: categorization and the experience of emotion. Personal. Soc. Psychol. Rev. **10**(1), 20–46 (2006)
11. Barrington, L., O'Malley, D., Turnbull, D., Lanckriet, G.: User-centered design of a social game to tag music. In: ACM SIGKDD, Paris, pp. 7–10 (2009)
12. Bingham, E., Mannila, H.: Random projection in dimensionality reduction: applications to image and text data. In: ACM SIGKDD, pp. 245–250 (2001)
13. Blitzer, J., Dredze, M., Pereira, F.: Biographies, Bollywood, boom-boxes and blenders: domain adaptation for sentiment classification. In: ACL, vol. 7, pp. 440–447 (2007)
14. Bradford Cannon, W.: Bodily Changes in Pain, Hunger, Fear and Rage: An Account of Recent Researches into the Function of Emotional Excitement. Charles T. Branford Company, Boston (1915)
15. Broca, P.: Anatomie comparée des circonvolutions cérébrales: Le grand lobe limbique. Rev. Anthropol. **1**, 385–498 (1878)
16. Cahill, L., McGaugh, J.: A novel demonstration of enhanced memory associated with emotional arousal. Conscious. Cogn. **4**(4), 410–421 (1995)
17. Calvo, M., Nummenmaa, L.: Processing of unattended emotional visual scenes. J. Exp. Psychol. Gen. **136**, 347–369 (2007)

18. Calvo, R., D'Mello, S.: Affect detection: an interdisciplinary review of models, methods, and their applications. IEEE Trans. Affect. Comput. **1**(1), 18–37 (2010)
19. Cambria, E., Fu, J., Bisio, F., Poria, S.: AffectiveSpace 2: enabling affective intuition for concept-level sentiment analysis. In: AAAI, Austin, pp. 508–514 (2015)
20. Cambria, E., Gastaldo, P., Bisio, F., Zunino, R.: An ELM-based model for affective analogical reasoning. Neurocomputing **149**, 443–455 (2015)
21. Cambria, E., Huang, G.B., et al.: Extreme learning machines. IEEE Intell. Syst. **28**(6), 30–59 (2013)
22. Cambria, E., Hussain, A.: Sentic Computing: A Common-Sense-Based Framework for Concept-Level Sentiment Analysis. Springer, Cham (2015)
23. Cambria, E., Hussain, A., Durrani, T., Havasi, C., Eckl, C., Munro, J.: Sentic computing for patient centered application. In: IEEE ICSP, Beijing, pp. 1279–1282 (2010)
24. Cambria, E., Hussain, A., Havasi, C., Eckl, C.: SenticSpace: visualizing opinions and sentiments in a multi-dimensional vector space. In: Setchi, R., Jordanov, I., Howlett, R., Jain, L. (eds.) Knowledge-Based and Intelligent Information and Engineering Systems. Lecture Notes in Artificial Intelligence, vol. 6279, pp. 385–393. Springer, Berlin (2010)
25. Cambria, E., Livingstone, A., Hussain, A.: The hourglass of emotions. In: Esposito, A., Vinciarelli, A., Hoffmann, R., Muller, V. (eds.) Cognitive Behavioral Systems. Lecture Notes in Computer Science, vol. 7403, pp. 144–157. Springer, Berlin/Heidelberg (2012)
26. Cambria, E., Mazzocco, T., Hussain, A., Eckl, C.: Sentic medoids: organizing affective commonsense knowledge in a multi-dimensional vector space. In: Liu, D., Zhang, H., Polycarpou, M., Alippi, C., He, H. (eds.) Advances in Neural Networks. Lecture Notes in Computer Science, vol. 6677, pp. 601–610. Springer, Berlin (2011)
27. Cambria, E., Olsher, D., Kwok, K.: Sentic activation: a two-level affective commonsense reasoning framework. In: AAAI, Toronto, pp. 186–192 (2012)
28. Cambria, E., Olsher, D., Kwok, K.: Sentic panalogy: swapping affective commonsense reasoning strategies and Foci. In: CogSci, Sapporo, pp. 174–179 (2012)
29. Cambria, E., Poria, S., Bajpai, R., Schuller, B.: Senticnet 4: a semantic resource for sentiment analysis based on conceptual primitives. In: Proceedings of COLING 2016, the 26th International Conference on Computational Linguistics: Technical Papers, pp. 2666–2677. The COLING 2016 Organizing Committee, Osaka (2016). http://aclweb.org/anthology/C16-1251
30. Cambria, E., Rajagopal, D., Kwok, K., Sepulveda, J.: GECKA: game engine for commonsense knowledge acquisition. In: FLAIRS, pp. 282–287 (2015)
31. Cambria, E., Xia, Y., Hussain, A.: Affective commonsense knowledge acquisition for sentiment analysis. In: LREC, Istanbul, pp. 3580–3585 (2012)
32. Chaiken, S., Trope, Y.: Dual-Process Theories in Social Psychology. Guilford, New York (1999)
33. Chklovski, T.: Learner: a system for acquiring commonsense knowledge by analogy. In: K-CAP, pp. 4–12 (2003)
34. Cochrane, T.: Eight dimensions for the emotions. Soc. Sci. Inf. **48**(3), 379–420 (2009)
35. Csikszentmihalyi, M.: Flow: The Psychology of Optimal Experience. Harper Perennial, New York (1991)
36. Dalgleish, T.: The emotional brain. Nat. Perspect. **5**, 582–589 (2004)
37. Dalgleish, T., Dunn, B., Mobbs, D.: Affective neuroscience: past, present, and future. Emot. Rev. **1**, 355–368 (2009)
38. Damasio, A.: Looking for Spinoza: Joy, Sorrow, and the Feeling Brain. Harcourt, Inc., Orlando (2003)
39. Eckart, C., Young, G.: The approximation of one matrix by another of lower rank. Psychometrika **1**(3), 211–218 (1936)
40. Epstein, S.: Cognitive-experiential self-theory of personality. In: Millon, T., Lerner, M. (eds.) Comprehensive Handbook of Psychology, vol. 5, pp. 159–184. Wiley & Sons, Hoboken (2003)

41. Fauconnier, G., Turner, M.: The Way We Think: Conceptual Blending and the Mind's Hidden Complexities. Basic Books (2003)
42. Fontaine, J., Scherer, K., Roesch, E., Ellsworth, P.: The world of emotions is not two-dimensional. Psycholog. Sci. **18**(12), 1050–1057 (2007)
43. Frijda, N.H.: The laws of emotions. Am. Psychol. **43**(5), 349 (1988)
44. Gupta, R., Kochenderfer, M., Mcguinness, D., Ferguson, G.: Commonsense data acquisition for indoor mobile robots. In: AAAI, San Jose, pp. 605–610 (2004)
45. Hacker, S., von Ahn, L.: Matchin: eliciting user preferences with an online game. In: CHI, Boston, pp. 1207–1216 (2009)
46. Havasi, C.: Discovering semantic relations using singular value decomposition based techniques. Ph.D. thesis, Brandeis University (2009)
47. Havasi, C., Speer, R., Alonso, J.: ConceptNet 3: a flexible, multilingual semantic network for commonsense knowledge. In: RANLP, Borovets (2007)
48. Havasi, C., Speer, R., Holmgren, J.: Automated color selection using semantic knowledge. In: AAAI CSK, Arlington (2010)
49. Herdagdelen, A., Baroni, M.: The concept game: better commonsene knowledge extraction by combining text mining and game with a purpose. In: AAAI CSK, Arlington (2010)
50. Huang, G.B.: An insight into extreme learning machines: random neurons, random features and kernels. Cogn. Comput. **6**(3), 376–390 (2014)
51. Huang, G.B., Cambria, E., Toh, K.A., Widrow, B., Xu, Z.: New trends of learning in computational intelligence. IEEE Comput. Intell. Mag. **10**(2), 16–17 (2015)
52. Huang, G.B., Chen, L., Siew, C.K.: Universal approximation using incremental constructive feedforward networks with random hidden nodes. IEEE Trans. Neural Netw. **17**(4), 879–892 (2006)
53. Huang, G.B., Wang, D.H., Lan, Y.: Extreme learning machines: a survey. Int. J. Mach. Learn. Cybern. **2**(2), 107–122 (2011)
54. Huang, G.B., Zhou, H., Ding, X., Zhang, R.: Extreme learning machine for regression and multiclass classification. IEEE Trans. Syst. Man Cybern. Part B: Cybern. **42**(2), 513–529 (2012)
55. Hussain, A., Cambria, E.: Semi-supervised learning for big social data analysis. Neurocomputing **275**, 1662–1673 (2018)
56. James, W.: What is an emotion? Mind **34**, 188–205 (1884)
57. Kirkpatrick, L., Epstein, S.: Cognitive experiential self-theory and subjective probability: further evidence for two conceptual systems. J. Pers. Soc. Psychol. **63**, 534–544 (1992)
58. Krumhuber, E., Kappas, A.: Moving smiles: the role of dynamic components for the perception of the genuineness of smiles. J. Nonverbal Behav. **29**(1), 3–24 (2005)
59. Kuo, Y., Lee, J., Chiang, K., Wang, R., Shen, E., Chan, C., Hu, J.Y.: Community-based game design: experiments on social games for commonsense data collection. In: ACM SIGKDD, Paris, pp. 15–22 (2009)
60. Lanczos, C.: An iteration method for the solution of the eigenvalue problem of linear differential and integral operators. J. Res. Natl. Bur. Stand. **45**(4), 255–282 (1950)
61. Law, E., von Ahn, L., Dannenberg, R., Crawford, M.: Tagatune: a game for music and sound annotation. In: International Conference on Music Information Retrieval, Vienna, pp. 361–364 (2007)
62. Lazarus, R.: Emotion and Adaptation. Oxford University Press, New York (1991)
63. Ledoux, J.: Synaptic Self. Penguin Books, New York (2003)
64. Lee, H., Grosse, R., Ranganath, R., Ng, A.Y.: Unsupervised learning of hierarchical representations with convolutional deep belief networks. Commun. ACM **54**(10), 95–103 (2011)
65. Lenat, D., Guha, R.: Building Large Knowledge-Based Systems: Representation and Inference in the Cyc Project. Addison-Wesley, Boston (1989)
66. Lewis, M.: Self-conscious emotions: embarrassment, pride, shame, and guilt. In: Handbook of Cognition and Emotion, vol. 2, pp. 623–636. Guilford Press (2000)
67. Lewis, M., Granic, I.: Emotion, Development, and Self-Organization: Dynamic Systems Approaches to Emotional Development. Cambridge University Press, Cambridge (2002)

68. Lieberman, M.: Social cognitive neuroscience: a review of core processes. Ann. Rev. Psychol. **58**, 259–89 (2007)
69. Lin, Z., Hwee, T., Kan, M.Y.: A PDTB-styled end-to-end discourse parser. Nat. Lang. Eng. **20**, 151–184 (2012)
70. Lu, Y., Dhillon, P., Foster, D.P., Ungar, L.: Faster ridge regression via the subsampled randomized Hadamard transform. In: Advances in Neural Information Processing Systems, pp. 369–377 (2013)
71. Ma, H., Chandrasekar, R., Quirk, C., Gupta, A.: Page hunt: improving search engines using human computation games. In: SIGIR, Boston, pp. 746–747 (2009)
72. Maclean, P.: Psychiatric implications of physiological studies on frontotemporal portion of limbic system. Electroencephalogr. Clin. Neurophysiol. Suppl. **4**, 407–18 (1952)
73. Manning, C.: Part-of-speech tagging from 97% to 100%: is it time for some linguistics? In: Gelbukh, A. (ed.) Computational Linguistics and Intelligent Text Processing. Lecture Notes in Computer Science, vol. 6608, pp. 171–189. Springer, New York (2011)
74. Markotschi, T., Volker, J.: GuessWhat?! – Human intelligence for mining linked data. In: EKAW, Lisbon (2010)
75. Mehrabian, A.: Pleasure-arousal-dominance: a general framework for describing and measuring individual differences in temperament. Curr. Psychol. **14**(4), 261–292 (1996)
76. Menon, A.K., Elkan, C.: Fast algorithms for approximating the singular value decomposition. ACM Trans. Knowl. Discov. Data (TKDD) **5**(2), 13 (2011)
77. Minsky, M.: The Society of Mind. Simon and Schuster, New York (1986)
78. Minsky, M.: The Emotion Machine: Commonsense Thinking, Artificial Intelligence, and the Future of the Human Mind. Simon and Schuster, New York (2006)
79. Morrison, D., Maillet, S., Bruno, E.: Tagcaptcha: annotating images with captchas. In: ACM SIGKDD, Paris, pp. 44–45 (2009)
80. Mueller, E.: Commonsense Reasoning. Morgan Kaufmann, Amsterdam (2006)
81. Neisser, U.: Cognitive Psychology. Appleton Century Crofts, New York (1967)
82. Ohman, A., Soares, J.: Emotional conditioning to masked stimuli: expectancies for aversive outcomes following nonre-cognized fear-relevant stimuli. J. Exp. Psychol. Gen. **127**(1), 69–82 (1998)
83. Oneto, L., Bisio, F., Cambria, E., Anguita, D.: Statistical learning theory and ELM for big social data analysis. IEEE Comput. Intell. Mag. **11**(3), 45–55 (2016)
84. Osgood, C., May, W., Miron, M.: Cross-Cultural Universals of Affective Meaning. University of Illinois Press, Urbana (1975)
85. Pang, B., Lee, L.: Seeing stars: exploiting class relationships for sentiment categorization with respect to rating scales. In: ACL, Ann Arbor, pp. 115–124 (2005)
86. Papez, J.: A proposed mechanism of emotion. Neuropsychiatry Clin Neurosci. **7**, 103–112 (1937)
87. Park, H., Jun, C.: A simple and fast algorithm for k-medoids clustering. Expert Syst. Appl. **36**(2), 3336–3341 (2009)
88. Plutchik, R.: The nature of emotions. Am. Sci. **89**(4), 344–350 (2001)
89. Poria, S., Cambria, E., Winterstein, G., Huang, G.B.: Sentic patterns: dependency-based rules for concept-level sentiment analysis. Knowl.-Based Syst. **69**, 45–63 (2014)
90. Rajagopal, D., Cambria, E., Olsher, D., Kwok, K.: A graph-based approach to commonsense concept extraction and semantic similarity detection. In: WWW, Rio De Janeiro, pp. 565–570 (2013)
91. Ridella, S., Rovetta, S., Zunino, R.: Circular backpropagation networks for classification. IEEE Trans. Neural Netw. **8**(1), 84–97 (1997)
92. Sarlos, T.: Improved approximation algorithms for large matrices via random projections. In: FOCS, pp. 143–152 (2006)
93. Scherer, K., Shorr, A., Johnstone, T.: Appraisal Processes in Emotion: Theory, Methods, Research. Oxford University Press, Canary (2001)
94. Siorpaes, K., Hepp, M.: Ontogame: weaving the semantic web by online games. In: ESWC, Tenerife, pp. 751–766 (2008)

95. Smith, E., DeCoster, J.: Dual-process models in social and cognitive psychology: conceptual integration and links to underlying memory systems. Personal. Soc. Psychol. Rev. **4**(2), 108–131 (2000)
96. Socher, R., Perelygin, A., Wu, J.Y., Chuang, J., Manning, C.D., Ng, A.Y., Potts, C.: Recursive deep models for semantic compositionality over a sentiment treebank. In: EMNLP, pp. 1642–1654 (2013)
97. Speer, R.: Open Mind Commons: an inquisitive approach to learning commonsense. In: Workshop on Commonsense and Interactive Applications, Honolulu (2007)
98. Speer, R., Havasi, C.: ConceptNet 5: a large semantic network for relational knowledge. In: Theory and Applications of Natural Language Processing (2012)
99. Speer, R., Havasi, C., Lieberman, H.: Analogyspace: reducing the dimensionality of commonsense knowledge. In: AAAI (2008)
100. Strapparava, C., Valitutti, A.: WordNet-affect: an affective extension of WordNet. In: LREC, Lisbon, pp. 1083–1086 (2004)
101. Thaler, S., Siorpaes, K., Simperl, E., Hofer, C.: A survey on games for knowledge acquisition. Tech. rep., Semantic Technology Institute (2011)
102. Tracy, J., Robins, R., Tangney, J.: The Self-Conscious Emotions: Theory and Research. The Guilford Press, New York (2007)
103. Tropp, J.A.: Improved analysis of the subsampled randomized Hadamard transform. Adv. Adapt. Data Anal. **3**(01n02), 115–126 (2011)
104. Tversky, A.: Features of similarity. Psychol. Rev. **84**(4), 327–352 (1977)
105. Vogl, T.P., Mangis, J., Rigler, A., Zink, W., Alkon, D.: Accelerating the convergence of the back-propagation method. Biol. Cybern. **59**(4-5), 257–263 (1988)
106. Westen, D.: Implications of developments in cognitive neuroscience for psychoanalytic psychotherapy. Harv. Rev. Psychiatry **10**(6), 369–73 (2002)
107. Yan, J., Yu, S.Y.: Magic bullet: a dual-purpose computer game. In: ACM SIGKDD, Paris, pp. 32–33 (2009)
108. Zeki, S., Romaya, J.: Neural correlates of hate. PLoS One **3**(10), 35–56 (2008)
109. van Zwol, R., Garcia, L., Ramirez, G., Sigurbjornsson, B., Labad, M.: Video tag game. In: WWW, Beijing (2008)

Chapter 4
Application to Sentiment Analysis

Abstract This chapter illustrates the building and expansion of WordNet for Medical Events (WME) and evaluate its performance. WME has been developed for medical opinion mining and can be used as a standalone medical lexicon. ConceptNet has been used to improve the graphical representation of the underlying architecture in WME. Two methods have been proposed and incorporated to improve the overall performance of the lexicon. First method adds two new features to the existing WME namely affinity and gravity score. To evaluate the new structure, machine learning techniques and linguistic approaches have been incorporated. Finally, the chapter proposes a novel fusion of computational creativity and machine learning.

Keywords WordNet for medical events • Affinity score • Gravity score • ConceptNet • Hybrid approach • Medical lexicon • Computational creativity • K-means

In the process of preparing the sentiment or opinion based medical lexicon, the current research aims to not only enrich the existing knowledge-base with additional concepts but also to extract more knowledge-based and sense-based features from the internet. The results in this chapter are aimed at preparing sentiment-oriented concept clusters with the addition of semantics and affinity features. We have introduced gravity as a feature to justify the relevance of the medical concepts and their respective glosses (glosses are the summary or definition of the medical term). Gravity depicts the degree of relatedness between the medical concepts/words and their gloss. The probabilistic-based approach has been used to calculate the affinity and gravity score of the medical concepts. In this process, the hybrid approach involving linguistics and machine learning have been introduced to evaluate the performance of the proposed WME structure. The fundamental aim of this research is to set up the WME as a lexical resource for medical sentiment or opinion analysis.

4.1 Sentiment Extraction from Medical Concepts

The knowledge-based sentiment lexicon is crucial in designing a context based sentiment extraction system. The medical concepts and their linguistic features are

© Springer International Publishing AG 2017
R. Satapathy et al., *Sentiment Analysis in the Bio-Medical Domain*,
Socio-Affective Computing 7, https://doi.org/10.1007/978-3-319-68468-0_4

extracted from the domain-specific sentiment lexicon. To overcome the problem
of experts availability, WME2.0 lexicon is formulated with a hybrid approach. It
adds an additional dimension in order to improve the accuracy of the extracted
medical context sentiment. The proposed hybrid approach [7] is the combination
of linguistic and machine learning approach. The approach consists of two phases
namely preprocessing Sect. 4.1.1 and learning phase in Sect. 4.1.2.

4.1.1   Preprocessing Phase

The preprocessing phase extracts the sentiments of medical contexts in the form of
context related medical concepts, their sentiments, and knowledge-based information. The structured form of the concepts are essential in identifying the important
medical concepts from the context. In this concern, to convert the unstructured
data into structured three steps were followed. The research community has
provided various open-source data preprocessing tools, for example, NLTK [4] as
linguistic resources which were introduced in the proposed hybrid algorithm as well.
Figure 4.1 shows the architecture of the proposed approach. The following steps
illustrate the basic operations of the preprocessing phase:

1. **Data Extraction**: The primary responsibility of this step is to extract the medical
   concepts from a given context. WME2.0 helps to extract the medical concepts

Fig. 4.1 Sentiment
Extraction Phases (Source:
[7])

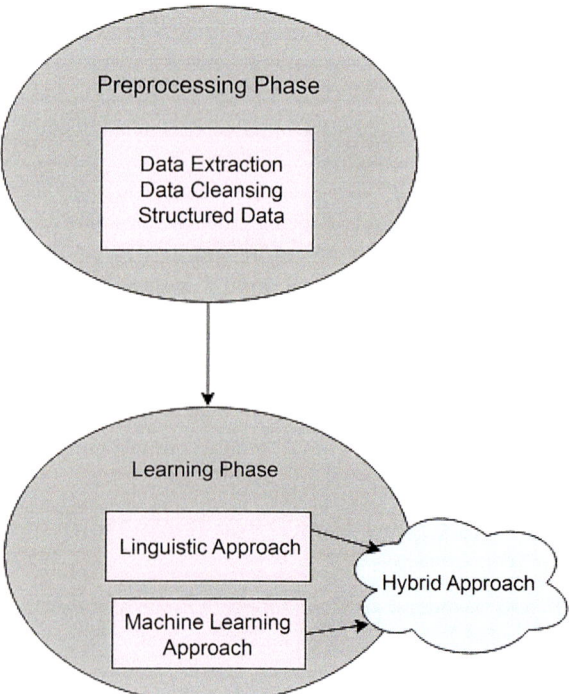

and their linguistic and sense-based features from the context. Moreover, the non-medical concepts/words and their sense identification are also essential to identify the sentiment of the context. The non-medical concepts and words related senses have been extracted using SenticNet lexicon [2] and SentiWord-Net [1] respectively.

2. **Data Cleansing:** This step removes the context related stop-words and concepts are stemmed. The classification of medical and non-medical words and identification of negation words such as no, not, never etc. are also taken care in the data cleansing step. Hence, a negating word like no, not or never changes the polarity of all the subsequent concepts as shown in Fig. 4.3. Figure 4.2 depicts the procedure followed for positive sentiment extraction.

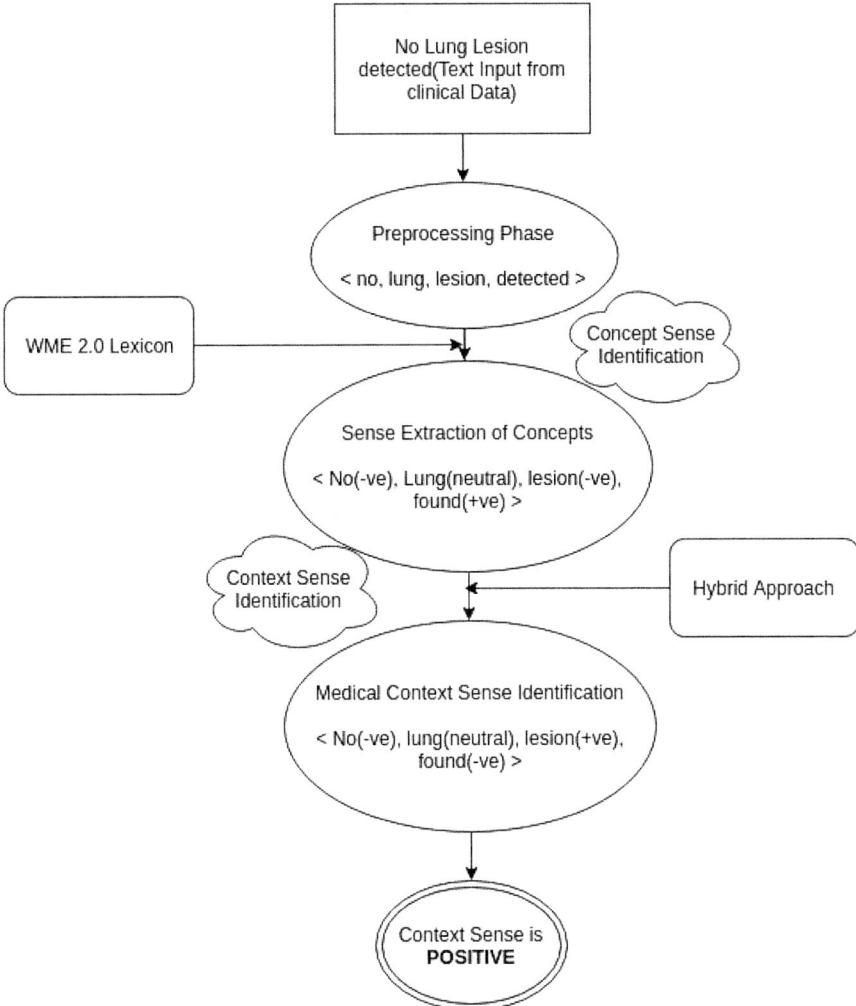

Fig. 4.2 Positive Sentiment extraction (Source: [7])

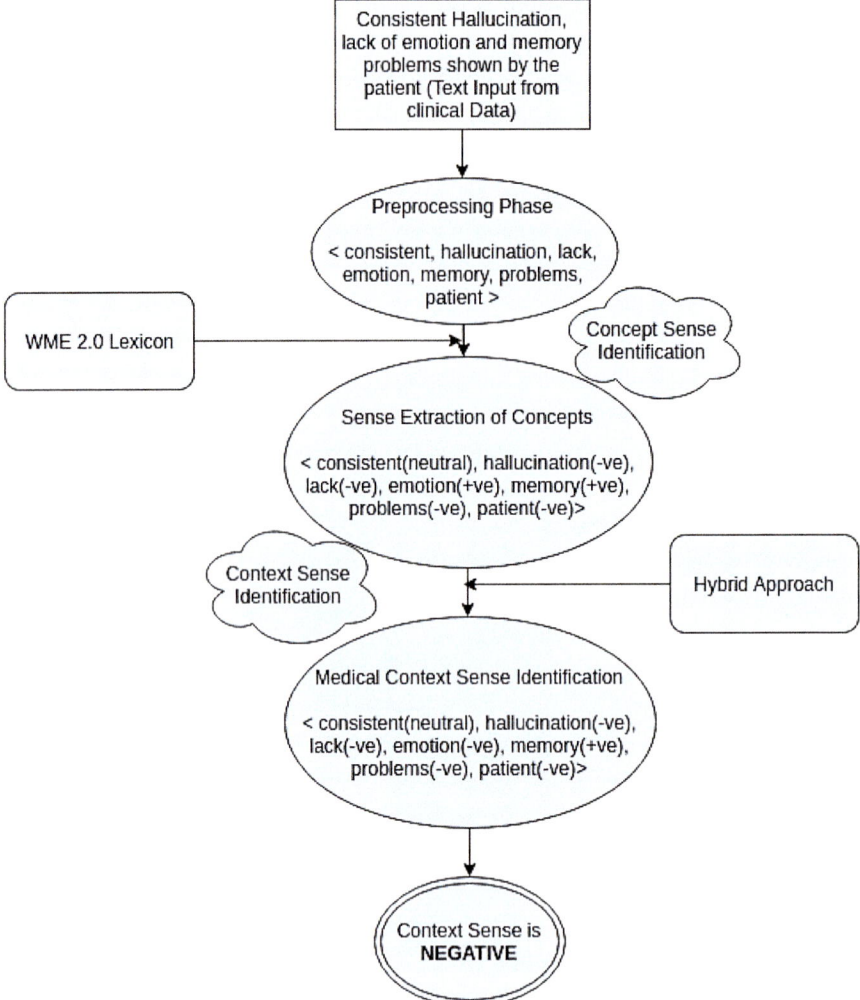

Fig. 4.3 Negative Sentiment extraction (Source: [7])

3. **Data Formatting:** Data formatting has been applied to represent the structured form of the extracted medical concepts. The extracted structured words (vectors) have been forwarded to the learning phase along with their features. The concept structure is represented as follows:

⟨ Concept(gastric), POS(noun), Semantics (abdominal breathing,visceral, intestinal,belly, duodenal,stomachic), Polarity Score(-0.5), Sense(Negative) ⟩

4.1.2 Learning Phase

Followed by the preprocessing phase, machine learning and linguistic methods were incorporated to extract the sentiments. The linguistic features and knowledge-based WME2.0 lexicons help to extract the hidden rules to understand the overall sentiment of the context. The context is accompanied with the polarity score and sense of each concept. The linguistic approach based extracted rules are fed to the supervised machine learning classifiers to evaluate the accuracy of the model. The linguistic approach is built so as to handle the negation effect in the context which helps to recognize the appropriate sense of the context. The algorithm for the learning phase is illustrated as follows:

Algorithm 4.1: The algorithm for the Learning Phase

Result: $Context_{polarity}$
$Context_{polarity} = 0$;
while *End of Line* **do**
    if *negation word* **then**
        Handle negation using linguistic approach;
    end
    Calculate Polarity of each concept/word;
    $Context_{polarity} = \sum_N Polarity_c$; where N = number of concept in the context
    and $Polarity_c$ indicates the polarity score of the concept.
end

The algorithm takes the medical text as input and provides the polarity score of the overall text as output.

4.2 Extending WME

WME is a free-standing lexical database [6] for researchers of NLP in the medical domain. It tries minimizing knowledge gap between doctors and patients. The WME was built with the aim of not only representing medical concepts for experts and non-experts but also to serve as a platform to review and validate the medical corpus. The experts can identify and extract the medical concepts and their corresponding definitions and descriptions. The non-experts can avail the WME lexicon to understand generic medical information since the concepts present in WME are validated based on the context and polarity. Polarity detection is a popular NLP task focusing on the binary classification of snippets of text into either positive or negative. Two new features namely: affinity Sect. 4.2.1 and gravity Sect. 4.2.2 were added to the existing lexicon to make the lexicon more stable with statistical significance added to it.

4.2.1   Affinity Score Spotting

Affinity refers to the link between the medical concepts in terms of their semantic relatedness. Affinity score calculates the degree of semantic relatedness of the medical concepts. Using the affinity scores of the concepts; concept clusters can be built by determining how different concepts are linked to each other in terms of their degree of semantic relatedness. The concept clusters are important for the building of a concept network that ensures better visualization of the concepts by seeing how they are associated with each other semantically. For example, the medical concept "brain" has affinity score of 0.290 for "alive"; 0.1540 for "clog" and 0.0560 for "fall in love" which indicates the degree of relatedness between these concepts. The numbers depend on the corpora used to calculate the affinity. Affinity score is calculated using probabilistic-based measurements. The concept's affinity ($Affinity_c$) calculates the degree of relationship between two words by measuring the number of semantic features they have in common. Equation 4.1 shows the process of computing $Affinity_c$.

$$Affinity_c = Sem_{MC_1} \cap Sem_{MC_2} \tag{4.1}$$

where Sem_{MC_1} and Sem_{MC_2} represents the semantics of the two different medical words. Example: MC_1 = 'brain' and MC_2 = 'limb'

The extracted affinity ($Affinity_c$) is then used to determine the Affinity score ($Affinity\text{-}Score_c$) of these words by using Eq. 4.2

$$Affinity - -Score_c = Affinity_c / \sum_{i=1}^{N} MC_i \tag{4.2}$$

where N is the number of medical concepts given as input; $Affinity\text{-}Score_c$ provides the co-reference relation between these medical concepts. Additionally, the $Affinity\text{-}Score_c$ of the concepts is derived from the semantic polarity and sense-based features of the concepts. $Affinity\text{-}Score_c$ has values that vary from 0 to 1; where 0 represents no relation between the medical concepts and 1 represents exactly similar medical concepts. In Fig. 4.4, we have illustrated the procedure in calculating the affinity score of the medical concepts.

4.2.2   Gravity Score Spotting

Gravity is essential for identifying the sentiment-oriented features such as polarity, sense and semantic features of the concepts in the gloss. It gives a deeper understanding of the concept senses in relation to their context of use. Gravity score provides the level of usefulness of the gloss or contextual information pertaining to a medical concept, which can be manually fine-tuned if it is too low. Gravity approach enhances the WME resource by providing a mean to emulate the human thought

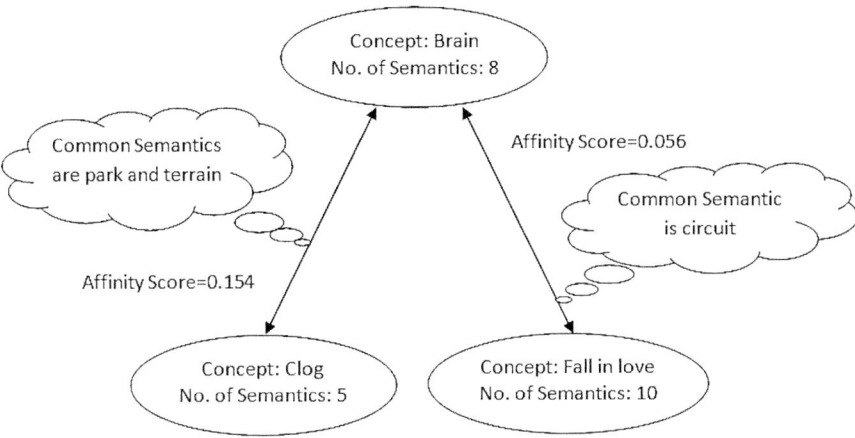

Fig. 4.4 Affinity Score Detection (Source: [5])

process in the recommendation of medical advice. It also serves as a foundation to build systems that model higher-order cognitive processes such as natural language processing.

In this research, the glosses of the medical concepts have been extracted from several knowledge-based resources. Gravity feature has been introduced to justify the relation between the concept and its respective gloss. Gravity score is calculated by measuring the polarity score differences between the concept and its gloss as shown in Eq. 4.3.

$$Gravity_c = Polarity_{gloss} - Polarity_c/N \qquad (4.3)$$

where $Gravity_c$ indicates the gravity score of the concept's gloss, $Polarity_c$ shows the polarity score of the concept while $Polarity_{gloss}$ represents the polarity score of the gloss of the concept. 'N' is the normalizing factor which stands for the number of words in the gloss. In other words, we can call $Gravity_c$ as the weight difference between the gloss polarity and concepts' polarity averaged over a number of words. After calculating the gravity score for each of the words that form the gloss of the respective concept, the final gravity score is computed in Eq. 4.4.

$$Gravity - Score_c = \sum_{i=1}^{N} Gravity_{c_i} \qquad (4.4)$$

where $Gravity\text{-}Score_c$ indicates the final gravity score that shows the relation of the concept with the gloss of the concept and N is the number of words in the gloss. Considering the medical concept *broadcloth* and its gloss as *a densely textured woolen fabric with a lustrous finish*, then the gravity score is 0.280 for the above-mentioned concept. Gravity score has values that vary on a three-point scale from

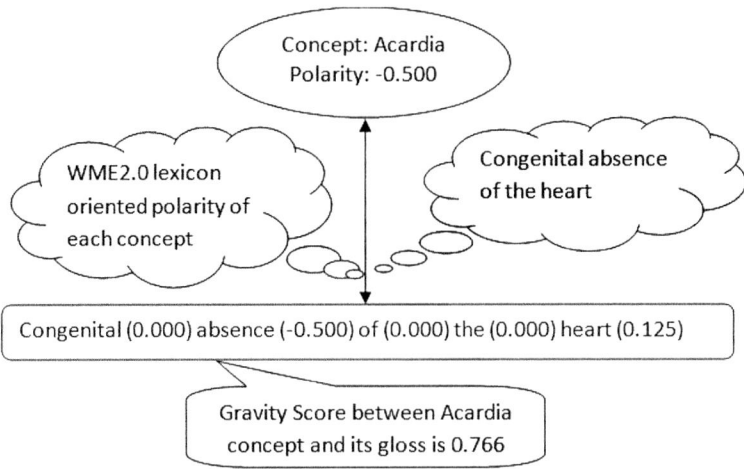

Fig. 4.5 Gravity Score Detection (Source: [5])

−1 to 1, where −1 represents a complete denial of gloss polarity with the concept's and 1 represents a complete agreement between the gloss and the concept. Figure 4.5 describes the gravity score retrieval procedure in detail.

4.2.3 Evaluation

The dataset is in a vector form: ⟨ Concept, Gloss, Affinity, Gravity, Polarity ⟩. Each row represents the medical concepts. Medical concepts were extracted from MedicineNet.[1]

4.2.3.1 Linguistic Approach

It is difficult to identify the syntactical or POS-based features of the medical concepts when they are extracted from the corpus due to the unstructured nature of the medical corpora and lack of involvement from the domain experts. The use of sentiment or opinion lexicons like SenticNet[2] and SentiWordNet[3] are also not effective to perform accuracy analysis on the medical concepts due to the paucity of medical words in these databases. For this reason, WME has to be utilized to overcome the difficulty of using lexical and/or syntactical analysis. To resolve

---

[1]http://www.medicinenet.com

[2]http://www.sentic.net/api/

[3]http://www.sentiwordnet.isti.cnr.it/

this difficulty and identify the accuracy of WME lexicon, sense-based approaches were utilized in this research. Unfortunately, there are no existing sentiment or opinion-oriented lexicons that are specifically targeted to the medical domain, so conventional sentiment or opinion resources like SentiWordNet, SenticNet, Bing Liu and Taboada Adjective list have to be used. These conventional sentiment lexicons along with English Medical Dictionary was compared against the medical concepts and their features by agreement analysis so as to calculate the lexical accuracy of WME. The agreement analysis was conducted by two manual annotators, and the verification output for the concepts has been provided in form of "yes" and "no". Under the agreement analysis, the first annotator labeled 6415 concepts as "yes" and 270 concepts as "no", while the second annotator gave 6171 concepts as "yes" and "244" concepts as "no". Between them, they have commonly agreed 6094 concepts as "yes" and 193 concepts as "no". From these tabulations, the agreement score was evaluated using CohenâĂŹs kappa statistical approach [11]. The following Eq. 4.5 calculates the kappa (κ) value from the Proportionate (Pr(a)) and Random (Pr(e)) agreement scores.

$$\kappa = [Pr(a) - Pr(e)]/[1 - Pr(e)] \qquad (4.5)$$

where, Pr(a) is the relative observed agreement among raters, and Pr(e) is the hypothetical probability of chance agreement, using the observed data to calculate the probabilities of each observer randomly saying each category. If the raters are in complete agreement then $\kappa = 1$. If there is no agreement among the raters other than, what would be expected by chance (as given by Pr(e)), $\kappa \leq 0$. After considering linguistic and knowledge-based features, the system has achieved a 0.73 κ score that indicates a satisfactory accuracy for the WME2.0. Kappa Score is a statistical approach which measures inter-rater agreement for categorical items. In other words, Cohen's kappa measures the agreement between two raters who each classify 'N' different items into 'C' mutually exclusive categories. It is generally thought to be a more robust measure than simple percent agreement calculation, since κ removes the possibility of the agreement occurring by chance as well.

4.2.3.2 Machine Learning Approach

Machine Learning was used in addition to Linguistic approach for the evaluation of the lexicon built. The K-Means classifier provides the F-Measure score against the distribution of the dataset. The distribution of dataset and F-Measure score are illustrated in Tables 4.1 and 4.2. Under the K-Means classifier approach, the table above indicates that the average F-Measure score of the WME2.0 resource is 0.974. In contrast, the Naïve Bayes and SMO supervised classifiers calculated the F-Measure score with four different approaches, namely use training set, supplied test set, Cross-validation Folds 10 and Percentage split %66. Tables 4.3 and 4.4 indicates the F-Measure score of these supervised classifiers by using the Naïve Bayes and SMO supervised classifiers approach.

Table 4.1 K-Means
unsupervised classifier for
WME v2.0 (Source: The
Authors)

Training(%)	Test(%)	F-Measure
85	15	0.992
80	20	0.996
75	25	0.993
70	30	0.974
65	35	0.995
60	40	0.961

Table 4.2 K-Means
unsupervised classifier for
WME v1.0 (Source: The
Authors)

Training(%)	Test(%)	F-Measure
85	15	0.891
80	20	0.887
75	25	0.884
70	30	0.875
65	35	0.896
60	40	0.856

Table 4.3 F-Measure of
Supervised classifiers for
WME v1.0 (Source: The
Authors)

Model	Naïve bayes	SMO
Supplied test set	0.915	0.915
Cross-validation Folds 10	0.964	0.967
Percentage split %66	0.973	0.979

Table 4.4 F-Measure of
Supervised classifiers for
WME v2.0 (Source: The
Authors)

Model	Naïve bayes	SMO
Supplied test set	0.815	0.815
Cross-validation Folds 10	0.864	0.867
Percentage split %66	0.853	0.854

After taking the approaches into consideration, the supplied test set model was used for measuring the sentiment oriented accuracy of the lexicon. Finally, the accuracy score from the machine learning approach was noted to be 91% for the WME2.0 lexicon resource in contrast to 80% in WME1.0. Clearly, addition of new features and concepts has led to a huge increase in performance parameters.

4.3 Medical Concept Network (MediConceptNet) Preparation

Incorporating concept network into WME promises to leverage better visualisation of the medical related sentiment knowledge. The MediConceptNet identifies the concepts and their sense related information using WME2.0 lexicon. The lexicon incorporates 6415 (It includes both diseases and symptoms) number of medical concepts along with Part-of-Speech (POS), gloss of the concept, semantics, polarity, sense and affinity features. In this section Graphical user Interface (GUI) for WME has been incorporated on top of WME lexicon. It is prepared with network models on top of the WME resource in order to assist the extraction of relational knowledge of these concept in a more user-friendly manner.

4.3.1   Semantic Network (SemNet) Preparation

For extracting the proper knowledge from the medical context, the sentiment or opinion related information is essential. SenticNet, SentiWordNet, Bing Liu opinion lexicons along with dictionaries, ontologies and WordNet [3] are taken into account to identify the sentiment based knowledge from the corpus. The WordNet or ontology based approaches helps to retrieve the synonyms, hyponyms and antonyms of the concept whereas the sentiment lexicon justifies the relevance of these retrieved concepts against sentiment. These ontology approaches are focused on expanding the lexical resources along with knowledge-based concepts. These knowledge and sentiment oriented lexicons are not that easy to understand. Hence, having a GUI could help people understand in a better way. In this concern, the visualization effect related to the concept sense based knowledge extraction approach was done. The WME medical lexicon and its probability directed affinity feature assists to develop a visualization system to better understand the concept and related sense knowledge information. The semantics extracted from WME of a concept are represented under Semantic Network (SemNet) with an affinity score ranging from 0 to 1. The affinity score of 1 indicates the full-relation between the concept and the semantics. The SemNet helps to understand pictorially the group of medical concepts with same sense knowledge bases. These concept cluster helps us in preparing Medical Concept Network framework with single concept networks (Fig. 4.6) and paired concept networks (Fig. 4.7).

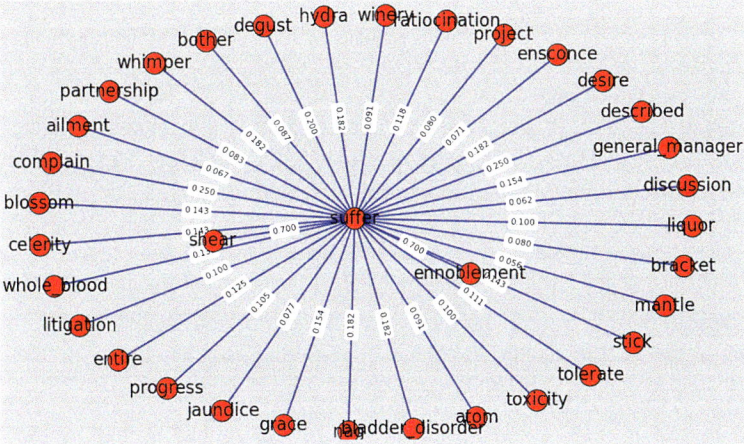

Fig. 4.6 Single Concept Conceptnet (Source: [5])

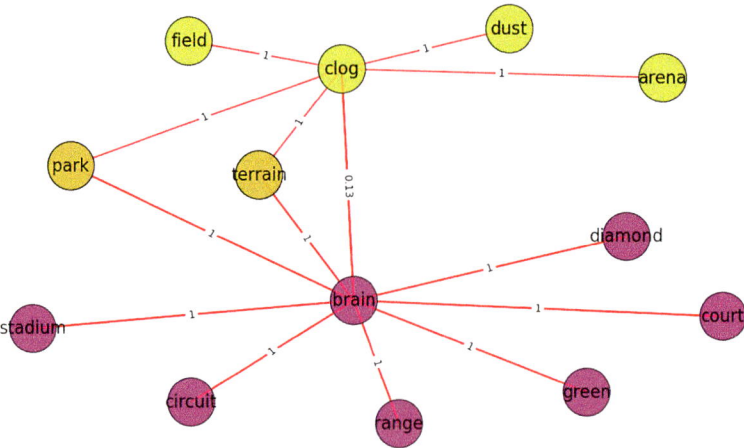

Fig. 4.7 Paired-concept Network (Source: [5])

These networks display the feasibility to extract quality commonsense knowledge from the medical context under MediConceptNet. Here, the relation between
the two concepts are extracted and represented using our GUI. The weight on
the edges of the graph shows the degree of similarity Sect. 4.2.1 between two
concepts. Two types of concept networks has been presented under MediConceptNet framework known as single-concept network and paired-concept network.
The single-concept network represents graphically all possible partial-relation
constructed concepts of a given medical concept. On the other side the paired-
concept network represents the relationship between two different medical concepts
which could either be partial, no or full relation. The single-concept network
indicates the general sentimental knowledge base information of the particular
concept where paired-concept network looks into inter concept relation which is for
specific sense oriented relations between these medical concepts. Figures 4.6 and 4.7
shows the representation technique of single-concept and paired-concept network
under WME2.0 respectively. These networks display the feasibility to extract quality
commonsense knowledge from the medical context under MediConceptNet. The
sense based full-relation along with no-relation and partial-relation of the concept
graph is the core to the MediConceptNet. No-relation graph indicates that there is no
sense or knowledge-based relation between the concepts whereas the partial-relation
indicated that for few semantics the concepts are related. The graphical based
concepts' information helps to develop more applications which are not restricted
to text document but also to different forms of natural languages. The proposed
sense based medical concept network framework has been developed by the 6415
number of medical concepts of WME2.0 lexicon. These number of concepts and
their related syntactic and sentiment features represented as XML format which
enriches to represent the semantic clusters under Bio-NLP domain. The sense and
polarity of a concept represents the commonsense knowledge-based information of
the concept.

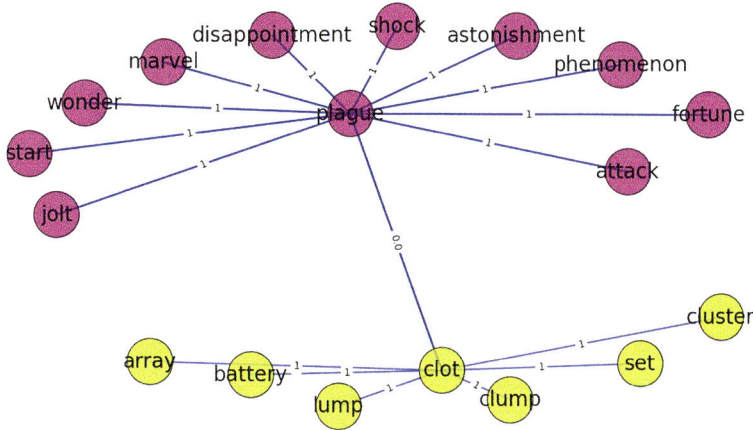

Fig. 4.8   No-relation based MediConceptNet (Source: [5])

Among all these properties the polarity, sense, and semantics of the medical concept have been represented as a vector for further steps. The "abdominal breathing" concept is represented as ⟨ '-0.5', 'Negative', 'visceral, intestinal, belly, gastric, duodenal, stomachic' ⟩.

The vector indicates the sense and knowledge-based information which matches/aligns with the primary concept of the vector. This above-mentioned mapping logic aids to build the semantic network (SemNet).

The sense based full-relation along with no-relation and partial-relation of the concept helps to build the MediConceptNet. No-relation indicated do not have any sense or knowledge-based relation present between the concepts whereas the partial-relation indicates few cases these concepts are related. Affinity score helps to justify the weight on the edges. The affinity score calculates the probability of occurrences of commonsense based semantics between two concepts. Now, the Figs. 4.8 and 4.9 shows the representation of no-relation and full-relation established in MediConceptNet respectively. The MediConceptNet Graphical User Interface (GUI) has been designed to consolidate all possible affinity as discussed in Sect. 4.2.1 through sense directed knowledge graph under an umbrella.

4.3.2   Evaluation

To build a concept network, a domain-specific lexicon is essential with conceptual features of the concepts under NLP. This task is even more noticeable when the concern is to build a structured corpus in a specific domain. The aim is to develop an intelligent cognitive system in medical field using conceptual features like affinity, polarity scores and semantic with a visualization to make it user-friendly. The system helps to cluster similar sentiment base concepts and identify semantic

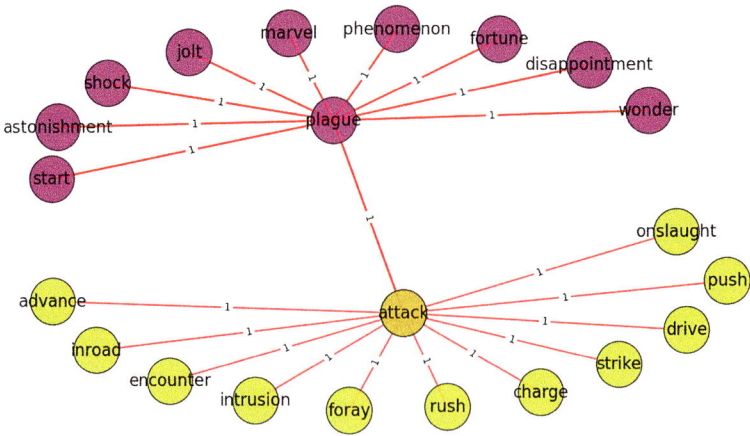

Fig. 4.9 Full-relation based MediConceptNet (Source: [5])

```
<Concept>amnesia<\Concept>
<Properties>
<POS>noum<\POS>
<Gloss>
   loss of memory sometimes including the memory
   of personal identity due to brain injury, shock,
   fatigue, repression, or illness or sometimes
   induced by anesthesia.
<\Gloss>
<Semantic>memory_loss,blackout, fugue, stupor<\Semantic>
<Polarity_score>-0.375<\Polarity_score>
<Affinity_score>0.429<\Affinity_score>
<Gravity_score>0.170<\Gravity_score>
<Sense>negative<\Sense>
<\Properties>
```

Fig. 4.10 WME2.0 lexicon representation for a concept amnesia (Source: [5])

relations between medical concepts. To validate the proposed medical concept
network and its data under WME2.0 lexicon, we adopt an agreement analysis
due to lack of annotated data. The agreement analysis involves the annotated
statistics provided by medical practitioners. The human annotators contribute
validated medical concepts and their semantic relations based on their practical
experience and WME2.0 lexicon. The reason for considering WME2.0 lexicon as
a baseline system is due to the maximum presence of the medical concepts over
other sentiment lexicons. Conventionally well-known sentiment lexicons such as
SenticNet and SentiWordNet only consider 26% and 40% coverage of the medical
concepts presented in WME2.0, which are not effective to get the accuracy of
medical concepts due to the shortage of medical words (concepts) in these resources.
On the other hand, WME2.0 lexicon satisfies 10186 number of medical concepts in
total and their affinity score, gloss, gravity score, Parts Of Speech (POS), polarity
score, semantics, and sense features as shown in Fig. 4.10.

4.4   Computational Creativity and Machine Learning

Creative machines are an old idea, but only recently has computational creativity established itself as a research field with its own existence and research agenda. The goal of computational creativity research is to model, simulate and enhance creativity using computational methods. Data mining and machine learning can be used in a number of ways to help computers learn how to be creative, such as learning to generate new artifacts or to evaluate various qualities of newly created artifacts. Computational creativity is the use of computers and computational formalisms in the study of creativity. The language of computation, and specifically concepts like search, knowledge representation, algorithms, goals, and constraints, gives us a scientific framework with which to study phenomena related to creativity. It has been observed that creativity is a generative process in which the new knowledge that is generated describes the desired product. The generated product generally is either an artifact or an art, but in either case, it usually has to meet certain predefined (whether implicitly or explicitly) goals and constraints. In order to be considered a creative product the general harmony is that it has to have at least two properties:

1. It has to be novel; and
2. It has to be useful/valuable

While AI has showcased remarkable advances in the last decades and has reached maturity as a research field, on the other hand, its sibling, computational creativity, is in earlier phases of its development. Computational creativity can be characterized in a manner which is parallel to AI. Where AI studies how to execute assignments which would be deemed intelligent if performed by a human, computational creativity investigates performances which would be deemed creative if performed by a human. An example from real life is the design of a building. Usually, an architect begins by obtaining an explicit indication from the property owner/developer of what characteristics would be desired in the building (perhaps its height and other dimensions, intended use like commercial or residential etc.,). Implicit are additional constraints that have to be taken into account by the architect, such as satisfying the local building code, figuring out details that might influence design decisions (such as the type of subsoil in the intended building site, earthquake prone and the existence or non-existence of public transportation options nearby), etc. Eventually, the architect goes and does what architects do, and proposes a design for the building, but that isn't sufficient. If this design looks too much like many other buildings already in the locality, the architect won't be considered to be very creative. If the proposed design of the building looks interestingly different from all the buildings that previously existed but has no doors or other ways of getting in or out if built it wouldn't serve its purpose of being a building. Both novelty and usefulness have to be among the implicit constraints taken into account in order for the architect to produce designs that will be considered creative, and usually one limits the other. Making sure of achieving usefulness ensures that not too much novelty is present because even though a lack of novelty does not make for creative results, too much novelty seems to be something that people consider crazy rather than creative. There seems to be a trade-off between craziness and creativity. We don't want our AI systems to be crazy.

In general human designers are great at finding the right balance between these factors, and several algorithms have been proposed that allow the computer, or the computer in tandem with a human, to produce similar creative results, though often during the process many partially constructed proposed designs are eventually dumped because they just don't meet all of the initial objective and constraints, both explicit and implicit, in addition to finding the right balance between the criteria of novelty and usefulness. Machine learning is the tool computers use to generate new knowledge that wasn't explicitly available. The ways in which this new knowledge can be generated and the types of new knowledge that can be generated are varied, and a variety of different algorithms have been proposed over the years for different types of learning goals. One possible learning goal is to analyze a set of exemplars and find sub-groups of the exemplars. These sub-groups are what are known as clusters. Several clustering algorithms have been proposed that look at the original set of exemplars and try to identify patterns within them to help structure the set into interrelated subsets. Data mining and machine learning are here broadly understood as methods that analyze data and make useful discoveries or inferences from them. Such methods can be used in creative systems, e.g., to learn how to recognize desirable qualities in produced artifacts, or even to produce artifacts, helping these systems produce novel and valuable results. For instance, automatic analysis of Western pop music as in [8] could reveal patterns that can be used to generate fairly good imitations of the given music. Imitation, however, is just replication from different songs in a genre and is not really a creative act, and it is not the goal of computational creativity research.

An example from real life can be found when a person looks at the animals in an African savannah and starts noticing that some of them, but not all, have long necks, some of them, but not all, have vertical black and white stripes, some of them, but not all, are smaller and have curving horns, etc. If the person asks other people around about these things, it will become apparent that the others have also identified the same patterns (and have even labeled the first sub-group of animals "giraffes", the second group "zebras", and the third group "gazelles"). It's not that there aren't individual variations between giraffes (in fact the splotches of color on them are unique, like fingerprints in humans), but these variations are minor in comparison to the major differences between any giraffe and any of the non-giraffes in the savannah (the total height, the length of the neck, the gait, the coloring scheme). People are great at learning to cluster things in this way, and several algorithms have been proposed that allow the computer, or the computer in tandem with a human, to cluster too, though one of the things that have proven difficult to automate is the decision of how many clusters to look for.

Practical applications of computational creativity can be roughly categorized into two classes. The first class makes use of fully automatic creativity, e.g., in computer games to develop plots or to compose music on the fly, or as a part of human-machine communication in dialogue systems and conversational agents. Applications in the other class use creative techniques as components to support or enable human creativity, e.g., in music or advertising. Some of the most interesting applications will improve the usability and usefulness of various technological appliances and will support human creativity in different tasks, by creating "in new, unforeseen modalities that would be difficult or impossible for people".

In this section, we apply some ideas behind computational creativity to machine learning in order to propose a new way of deciding on the value for this parameter when performing clustering. In our work, clustering is treated as a generative method that proposes new knowledge that can be evaluated for its novelty and usefulness. Only the set of new clusters that represent the "best" combination of these two characteristics is ultimately learned, thus using ideas from computational creativity to inform our learning algorithm on how many clusters to look for.

4.4.1 Applications of Computational Creativity

Images have an important application in computational creativity field. While working with images in computational creativity, the first and foremost questions that come to our mind is: How do we produce images which look like a face? Or which expresses emotions like happiness or sadness? A popular and obvious choice then is to use genetic algorithms for generating candidate artifacts to be evaluated by classification or regression. In these cases, it is the fitness function eval(a) that is learned, while a genetic algorithm aims to implement the generation function gen() effectively by adapting to search for high-quality artifacts. The fitness of images is evaluated by a classifier trained to recognize if certain types of objects are present in the image. The evolutionary algorithm then tries to optimize the quality of produced images with respect to this evaluation (fitness) function. Applications of creativity are not limited to image generation or music generation. The use of regression to evaluate creative artifacts is illustrated by applications in quite a different field, cooking recipes. PIERRE [9], a computational stew recipe generator, first extracts different possible ingredients of stews, soups, and chilis from recipe websites. PIERRE then learns multiple multi-layer perceptrons on different levels of abstraction to model the relation between different recipes (essentially weighted combinations of ingredients) and the ratings given to the recipes on web sites. Then a genetic algorithm is used to generate recipes, evaluated using the learned perceptrons. A more elaborate cooking recipe generation system has been developed at IBM, considering the cultural context, physiochemical properties of flavor compounds, and even the name of the dish as components that influence the perception of flavors. The system uses many different machine learning techniques to extract information and to evaluate the quality of the produced recipes. In this section, we propose the combination of computational creativity and machine learning to calculate the novelty and usefulness of our proposed model on top of our designed dataset from Sect. 4.2. In the next Sect. 4.4.2 we describe how the WME data was prepared to apply computational creativity.

4.4.2   Source and Preparation of WME Data for Computational Creativity

To evaluate and measure the accuracy based disease and symptom clusters we [10] prepared the training and test datasets. The training dataset was prepared with the help of WME lexicon resource of medical concepts [6] which has 6415 concepts. We found 5066 diseases (we will use this term generically to refer to any identifiable medical condition) in WME. We prepared a matrix of associations between diseases and symptoms by using the 5066 diseases to consult two online engines, HealthLine Symptom Checker[4] and MedicineNet.[5] This allowed us to identify a total of 1149 different possible noise free symptoms.

Our next step was to identify semantics. These are diseases that appeared as different concepts in WME, yet are associated with exactly the same set of symptoms, so for computational purposes, they can be considered to be equivalent thereby decreasing our computation cost. Identifying synonyms allowed us to remove some noise from the data as well. For example: "HIV" and "human immunodeficiency virus" will have the same set of symptoms so these can be clustered together into one group. It can also be considered a preliminary version of clustering since it involves grouping together exemplars that were originally considered to represent different phenomena. This initial analysis allowed us to identify 3067 disease clusters; then the same method was on symptom set. Identifying similar symptoms means finding all those that are associated with the exact same set of diseases and found a total of 960 symptom clusters. For example, two of the original diseases, *mental depression* and *depressive disorder*, ended up being considered equivalent diseases, and have the same sets of symptoms: *suicidal tendencies, blackouts, weepiness, inability to concentrate, irritable mood, feeling hopeless* in the WME lexicon. Similarly, the *ritch* and *breath holding spell symptom* were clustered together in pattern based matching for the disease *gastroenteritis* (Fig. 4.11 and 4.12).

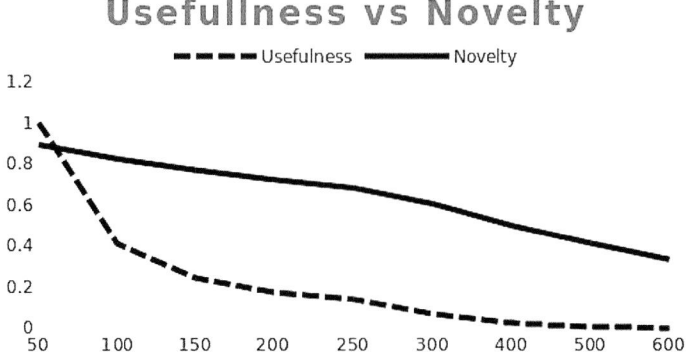

Fig. 4.11   Accuracy vs Novelty for Symptoms (Source: [10])

---

[4]http://www.healthchecker.com

[5]http://www.medicinenet.com

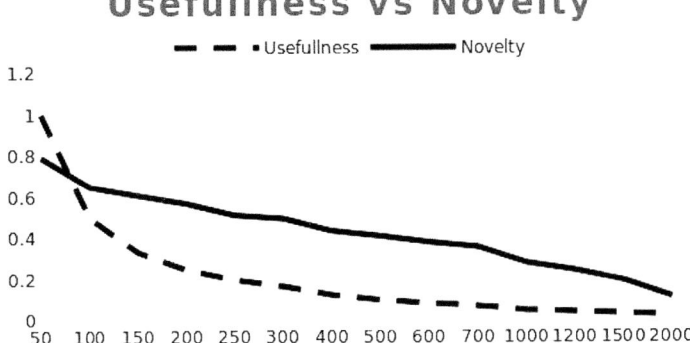

Fig. 4.12 Accuracy vs Novelty for Disease (Source: [10])

The performance of a given set of exemplars was measured by setting up a series of test problems or otherwise called queries. After obtaining the results of each individual query we averaged these results to find an overall measure of performance for the set of exemplars. In our case study, a query could consist of a symptom or a set of symptoms (in which case the output would be a set of possible diseases associated with these symptoms), or the query could be a disease or a set of diseases (in which case the output would be a set of possible symptoms associated with these diseases). First, the original set of diseases were analyzed and sorted them according to how many symptoms they were associated with. This helps to isolate those diseases that were associated with a relatively large set of symptoms. The top 500 diseases were taken as the rest values were negligible in order to consider only them in the generation of the test queries (and thus create tests with "common" diseases rather than outliers). We then created 250 test queries. For each test query, the number of diseases was chosen at random, and then that number of diseases was randomly chosen from the set of "top 500". Assuming that query Q1 consists of diseases D1, D2, and D3, then the result of the query would be the union of the sets of symptoms associated with each of D1, D2, and D3. If this set of diseases [D1, D2, D3] matches with two of the original symptom sets, S1 and S2, and we had 's' number of symptoms, then the performance of our data on this query would be $2/s$. In our measurements, the matching of a set of diseases to a given symptom is performed by determining whether the set of diseases is a subset of the diseases associated with that symptom, and this procedure is repeated for each candidate symptom. All of this by itself (i.e., for one query) would be a very rough estimate of the performance of our data, but after repeating the same procedure for 250 test queries and finding the mean performance, we have a more representative measure of performance (and just in case the 250 is thought to be arbitrary, we repeated the same procedure several times and obtained very similar results each time, which gives greater credence to the fact that the results that we have obtained are really representative). The above-mentioned cut-off for diseases and symptoms have been selected for proper justification of the original dataset and to reduce the test data redundancy. On the top of these diseases and symptoms, the random pattern generation process was applied with the random length test patterns. We can measure the accuracy of a given configuration of our data by comparing its performance (as defined above) with the performance of a base (reference) configuration on the same set of queries. For instance, if the performance of the original data is 5 and the performance of the same data but after having grouped together synonyms, on the same set of queries, is 50, then the accuracy of the data with synonyms compared to the original data is $50/5 = 10$. In this example, since the accuracy is above 1 there has been an improvement in performance after finding the synonyms. An accuracy value lower than 1 would represent a decrease in performance with respect to our base configuration. We have first prepared a test data set with 250 number of patterns (diseases and symptoms) to identify the performance and accuracy. The following steps followed to develop the test dataset:

1. Calculated the occurrences of the symptoms from the original dataset.
2. We have picked top 500 symptoms and diseases to prepare the test set.
3. On the top of these symptoms and diseases, we have run the random process to generate the random length test patterns.

After developing the test pattern, we have applied on the original dataset (5066 number of diseases and 1145 number of symptoms) to calculate the performance. In the case of pattern dataset (3067 number of diseases and 960 number of symptoms) and K-Means based datasets, the performance has been measured using the following algorithm:

Algorithm 4.2: Performance Measure is used as a measure to check the usefulness:

Result: Performance
    while *End of Test Patterns* **do**
        Compare test patterns with the generated clusters;
        if *Pattern match is Found* **then**
            Count the number of matches(k);
            Calculate k/n;
            Jump to the next test pattern;
        end
        Continue with the next set of test patterns;
        Performance $= \sum_{k=1}^{k=N}(k/n)/250$;
        Accuracy $= P_p / O_p$;
        where: P_p represents the Pattern or K-means dataset performance and O_p represents the Original dataset performance and 250 is the number of total test patterns generated and is used for normalization purpose.
    end

Fusing computation creativity with machine learning requires both novelty and usefulness to be present. Hence, the following points make a clear understanding of how the fusion is represented. The fusion of computation creativity and machine learning is the noble approach in the field of computation creativity.

1. Clustering step helps in getting new information in the form of clusters. Clusters are an indication that the disease and symptoms are similar not only semantically but syntactically as well.
2. To calculate how valuable the clustering is we proposed performance measure. It measures how good the clusters are doing on the test set provided by us.

The final Chap. 5 proposes a summary of contributions in terms of models, techniques, and tools.

References

1. Baccianella, S., Esuli, A., Sebastiani, F.: Sentiwordnet 3.0: an enhanced lexical resource for sentiment analysis and opinion mining. In: Proceeding of LREC (2010)
2. Cambria, E., Poria, S., Hazarika, D., Kwok, K.: SenticNet 5: discovering conceptual primitives for sentiment analysis by means of context embeddings. In: Proceedings of AAAI (2018)
3. Fellbaum, C.: WordNet: An Electronic Lexical Database. Language, Speech, and Communication. The MIT Press, Cambridge (1998)
4. Loper, E., Bird, S.: Nltk: the natural language toolkit. In: Proceedings of the ACL-02 Workshop on Effective Tools and Methodologies for Teaching Natural Language Processing and Computational Linguistics – Volume 1, ETMTNLP'02, pp. 63–70. Association for Computational Linguistics, Stroudsburg (2002)
5. Mondal, A., Cambria, E., Das, D., Bandyopadhyay, S.: Mediconceptnet: an affinity score based medical concept network. FLAIRS 335–340 (2017)
6. Mondal, A., Chaturvedi, I., Das, D., Bajpai, R., Bandyopadhyay, S.: Lexical resource for medical events: a polarity based approach. In: ICDM Workshops, pp. 1302–1309. IEEE (2015)
7. Mondal, A., Satapathy, R., Das, D., Bandyopadhyay, S.: A hybrid approach based sentiment extraction from medical context. In: 4th Workshop on Sentiment Analysis where AI meets Psychology (SAAIP 2016), IJCAI 2016 Workshop, Hilton, New York City, 10 July 2016 (2016)
8. Ni, Y., Santos-Rodriguez, R., Mcvicar, M., Bie, T.D.: Hit song science once again a science?
9. Pinel, F., Varshney, L.R.: Computational creativity for culinary recipes. In: CHI'14 Extended Abstracts on Human Factors in Computing Systems. ACM (2014)
10. de Silva Garza, A.G., Mondal, A., Satapathy, R.: Using computational creativity concepts to decide parameter values during clustering. In: Computing Conference, 2018
11. Viera, A., Garrett, J.: Understanding interobserver agreement: the kappa statistic. Fam. Med. **37**(5), 360–363 (2005)

Chapter 5
Conclusion and Future Work

Abstract The book gives an insight to Wordnet for Medical Events and applies commonsense computing and linguistic patterns to bridge the cognitive and affective gap between word-level medical data and the concept-level opinions conveyed by the medical contexts. This book introduces to a novel approach to decrease the gap between computational creativity and machine learning fields. This book also introduces to the microtext analysis which is an essential part for normalizing tweets and/or micro-blogs. This final section proposes a summary of contributions in terms of models, techniques and tools.

Keywords Opinion mining • Sentiment analysis • Biomedical text mining • Natural language processing • Deep learning • Sentic computing • WME

In order to develop a medical context sentiment extraction model, the important keyword extraction and their related sense and polarity score identification are crucial with semantic-based medical concept features. The statistical and linguistic features based medical sentiment lexicons are facing difficulty in Bio-NLP domain. Future works include the usage of WME as a module in the SenticNet, for handling the medical terms. With the rise of the internet, the real-time data are available for free. However, utilizing it for research is difficult as the grammar and vocabulary change from individual to individual. Hence, the importance of microtext analysis module comes into account. This book gives an introduction to microtext and its importance in the sentiment analysis task. The microtext analysis has a lot of application including cybercrime detection, terrorism spotting; machines will leverage on the lexicons and machine learning algorithms to interact with humans in future with the rise of AI. This can be extended to multiple languages [7] for sentiment analysis in biomedical domain. Furthermore, a dialogue system as in [9], can be built for biomedical domain so as to keep patients calm by chatting with them.

© Springer International Publishing AG 2017   127
R. Satapathy et al., *Sentiment Analysis in the Bio-Medical Domain*,
Socio-Affective Computing 7, https://doi.org/10.1007/978-3-319-68468-0_5

5.1   Summary of Contributions

Despite significant progress, opinion mining and sentiment analysis are still finding their own voice in new inter-disciplinary fields like biomedical domain and computation creativity. Hence, this book introduces to different applications of sentiment analysis with a main focus on the bio-medical domain. This book also introduces to the importance of a medical lexicon. It introduces WME which is a sense based medical lexicon. This book also introduces to a novel approach which fuses computational creativity and machine learning in the computational creativity field. The primary aim of the researchers is to build an intelligent automated system in the Bio-NLP domain, which can extract the unstructured knowledge-based information with proper sense and convert it to a structured one. Incorporating computational creativity with NLP could create new knowledge thereby decreasing the gap between humans and the machines. In this approach, the researchers have tried to incorporate computational creativity and machine learning.

5.1.1   Models

1. AffectNet: an affective commonsense representation model built by integrating different kinds of knowledge coming from multiple sources;
2. AffectiveSpace: a vector space model built by means of semantic multi-dimensional scaling (MDS) for reasoning by analogy on affective commonsense knowledge;
3. The Hourglass of Emotions: a biologically-inspired and psychologically- motivated model for the representation and the analysis of human emotions.
4. Hybrid Model for medical contexts: Inspired by linguists and machine learning experts, it tries to remove the limitations of medical contexts in machine learning.

5.1.2   Tools

1. SenticNet: a semantic and affective resource that assigns semantics and sentics with 50,000 concepts (also accessible through an API and a Python package);
2. WME: a medical context based lexicon that assigns polarity and sense-based information to the input text. It has 5066 diseases and 1149 different symptoms as a lexical resource.

5.2 Future Work

5.2.1 *Importance of Microtext Normalization*

Microtexts have become an important part of human's daily life. Many research works [1, 3–6] have tried to normalize it with different techniques. However, the question should be, do we need to spend so much time and effort on research to normalize it. Microtext can be treated as a new language and machines can be trained on the same. For example, when we deal with the Chinese language we don't always transform it into the English language. Languages use parallel corpora to train a machine learning system and learn the intrinsic features of a new language. As suggested in [8], a lot of research is going on in order to develop tools to attack the problem of Chinese language understanding as a standalone language and not just transforming it to English. In concept level we talk about sentic patterns, similarly, there are microtext patterns, which will remove the need of normalizing the microtexts. This approach will require lexicon, rule-based and deep learning all working together in order to achieve the goal. This will enhance human's capability to communicate with the machines using microtexts. AI as a concept was never existed to replace human effort, rather enhance it, because of AI's capability to make numerical faster than humans. Then humans taught machines the natural language in order to communicate with them. The actual problem here is why is microtext problem taken as a normalizing task and not as another language which most humans are pretty prominent with.

If machines could learn microtexts then the threats like terrorist attacks and piration of videos would be monitored easily and efficiently. It is high time for researchers to see microtext from a linguist perspective rather than just normalizing task.

5.2.2 *Public Health Measures*

In healthcare domain, it has long been recognized that, although a health professional is the adept in investigating, offering aid, and giving support in managing a clinical situation, the patient is the expert in living with that condition. However, there is a need to validate medical departments. The best contender for this is neither the doctor, the nurse, or the therapist, but the patient himself/herself. Patients, in fact, are usually keen on expressing their opinions and feelings in free text, especially if driven by particularly positive or negative emotions. They are often happy to share their healthcare experiences for different reasons, e.g., because they seek for a sense of togetherness in adversity, because they benefited from others' opinions and want to give back to the community, for cathartic complaining, for supporting a service they really like, because it is a way to express themselves, because they think their opinions are important for others. When people have a strong feeling about a specific service they utilized, they feel like expressing it. If they loved it, they want others to enjoy it. If they hated it, they want others to not go through the same.

Public health measures [2] such as better nutrition, greater access to medical care, improved sanitation, and more widespread immunization have produced a rapid decline in death rates across all age groups. Since there is no corresponding fall in birth rates, however, the average age of the population is increasing exponentially. If we want health services to keep up with such monotonic growth, we need to automatize as much as possible the way patients access the healthcare system, in order to improve both its service quality and timeliness. Everything we do that does not provide benefit to patients or their families, in fact, is a waste. The WME lexicon is built to provide the disease and symptom related queries. However, it lacks the nutrition-related concepts. WME needs to be enriched with the nutrition-related concepts so as to enable it to be used in every household. Symptoms, Diseases and Nutrition can be thought as a 3D matrix. This will help WME become a fully automated medical domain knowledge base which suggests nutrition for symptoms and diseases. Because the public does not only inquires about diseases related to their symptoms but also the nutrition which could help them curb the symptoms thereby putting their life back on track.

References

1. Beider, A.: Beider-Morse phonetic matching: an alternative to Soundex with fewer false hits. Avotaynu: The International Review of Jewish (2008)
2. Cambria, E., Benson, T., Eckl, C., Hussain, A.: Sentic PROMs: application of sentic computing to the development of a novel unified framework for measuring health-care quality. Expert Syst. Appl. **39**(12), 10533–10543 (2012)
3. Khoury, R.: Microtext Normalization using Probably- Phonetically-Similar Word Discovery. In: 2015 IEEE 11th International Conference on Wireless and Mobile Computing, Networking and Communications (WiMob), pp. 392–399 (2015)
4. Khoury, R., Khoury, R., Hamou-Lhadj, A.: Microtext Processing. Springer, New York (2014)
5. Kobus, C., Yvon, F., Damnati, G.: Normalizing SMS: are two metaphors better than one? In: Proceedings of the 22nd International Conference on Computational Linguistics, vol. 1, pp. 441–448. Association for Computational Linguistics (2008)
6. Li, C., Liu, Y.: Normalization of text messages using character-and phone-based machine translation approaches. INTERSPEECH, pp. 2330–2333 (2012)
7. Lo, S.L., Cambria, E., Chiong, R., Cornforth, D.: Multilingual sentiment analysis: from formal to informal and scarce resource languages. Artif. Intell. Rev. **48**(4), 499–527 (2017)
8. Peng, H., Cambria, E., Hussain, A.: A review of sentiment analysis research in Chinese language. Cogn. Comput. **9**(4), 423–435 (2017)
9. Young, T., Cambria, E., Chaturvedi, I., Zhou, H., Biswas, S., Huang, M.: Augmenting end-to-end dialogue systems with commonsense knowledge. In: Proceedings of AAAI (2018)

Index

© Springer International Publishing AG 2017
R. Satapathy et al., *Sentiment Analysis in the Bio-Medical Domain*,
Socio-Affective Computing 7, https://doi.org/10.1007/978-3-319-68468-0